Grow Your Practice Online

*Proven Strategies to Attract
and Convert New Dental Patients*

The Ultimate Guide to
Digital Marketing
for Your Dental Practice

Adam Zilko

Copyright © 2018 Adam Zilko

All rights reserved.

ISBN: 1986877035
ISBN-13: 978-1986877039

DISCLAIMER

The information contained in this book is based on real-life application and actual events, though some names have been changed for confidentiality reasons. We have put forth every effort to ensure that the information is accurate and complete. The information we present to you is designed to bring your dental practice all the success it can muster. However, due to variables beyond our control, such as your location and the state of current market conditions, we cannot be held responsible for any loss to your practice after this advice has been put into action. We sincerely hope that this advice works for you and we will do whatever we can to help.

A WORD ON THE TECHNOLOGIES AND TOOLS DISCUSSED IN THIS BOOK

Writing a book like this is tricky because we are describing technologies, tools, and processes that are used today, but that might not be valuable five or ten years from now. Therefore, we promise to make every effort only to mention the tools and techniques we feel will remain relevant long into the future. Furthermore, we will update these steps as necessary as new dental marketing methods are revealed to ensure you have the most advanced material to date.

CONTENTS

Preface 2

Chapter 1: Why Digital Excellence? 8

Chapter 2: Getting Your Mind Right for Digital Success 15

Chapter 3: Creating Your Digital Marketing "Treatment Plan" 29

Chapter 4: Make Conversions Your Focus 41

Chapter 5: The Marketing Funnel 52

Chapter 7: Dental Marketing Website Checklist 78

Chapter 8: An Introduction to Search Engine Optimization (SEO) 85

Chapter 9: Local Search Engine Optimization 110

Chapter 10: Staying Up-To-Date With Google 123

Chapter 11: Get on Facebook 128

Chapter 12: Reputation Management and Online Reviews 138

Chapter 13: Pay-Per-Click Search Engine Advertising 147

Chapter 14: Patient Retention & Reengagement 179

Chapter 15: Tracking, Testing & Troubleshooting Your Campaign 185

Conclusion - Where To Go From Here 197

Appendix 199

DO YOU HAVE QUESTIONS OR CONCERNS?

Contact us at Admin@Firegang.com.

The Dental Marketing Guide to Digital Excellence.

All rights reserved.

Copyright © 2018

Published by Firegang Dental Marketing

Written By: Adam Zilko

Edited By: Jason Little

ISBN-13: 978-1497462700

This book is protected under the copyright laws of the United States of America. Any reproduction or other unauthorized use of this material or the artwork contained herein is prohibited without the express written permission of the authors.

First Printing: April 2014

Printed in the United States of America

Second Edition: December 2014

Third Edition: December 2015

Fourth Edition: March 2018

DOWNLOAD THE BOOK BONUSES FREE!

As a thank you for purchasing our book, we would like to invite you to download the following free extra resources at www.firegang.com/book-bonuses/.

What you get:

- How to create "Next Level" Facebook ads

- Powerful scripts for most phone encounters (even price shoppers!)

- Tips to turn your front office into a goldmine

- How to protect and grow your online reputation

- Getting started with a Facebook Page – The Complete Guide

- Turn your website into a traffic converting machine

- Case Study: Multi-Location Practice Increases Patients by 30%!

Schedule your FREE consultation today to get all your questions answered. Call (800) 398-0979 or email sales-team@firegang.com. Or visit https://www.firegang.com/

PREFACE

A Note from Adam Zilko, Owner & Co-Founder of Firegang Dental Marketing

It has been a little over four years since the first edition of this book was published. A lot has happened in that short time. The world of dental marketing continues to accelerate at a breakneck pace, and my company - Firegang Dental Marketing – has, in turn, experienced massive growth.

Writing a book about digital marketing is quite a challenge. This is an industry that changes almost daily. New techniques rise to the fore while tried and true techniques – like backlinks after Panda – become blacklisted overnight.

While we made every effort to ensure that the previous book contained as much timeless information as possible, we knew needed to make some changes.

What follows is an up-to-date account of what it takes to make a dental practice successful using the most cutting-edge digital marketing techniques known today. We use these very techniques with our clients and offer step-by-step instructions on how to do the same for your practice.

Going Beyond Digital Marketing

One of our primary goals in writing this book was to stress the importance of the critical elements of digital marketing that can drastically affect your results, and that – believe it or not – have nothing to do with digital marketing at all.

We get it. You may think it silly to start a book about digital marketing with an aspect of your practice that has little to do about marketing, but we hope you'll soon realize just how essential these elements are.

We also want you to know that these factors are entirely within your control. However, unless they are correctly optimized, even if your digital marketing efforts are on point, you might be holding back your results.

These elements include mindset, office efficiency, patient service, and your reputation as a dental professional in your local community. For instance, you could have a website that attracts new patient leads in droves, but if your office staff can't close any appointments over the phone, your digital marketing efforts will be largely wasted.

Digital marketing is a comprehensive affair where every part must be optimized if you hope to earn a healthy return on your investment.

With this book as your guide, you will learn the very methods we teach to our clients to help them achieve their practice goals. Most importantly, you will learn how to treat your patients with the utmost respect and authority to make yours one of the most popular dental offices in town.

Building a successful dental practice is never easy, so I don't want to sugarcoat things. This is not something you can do all on your own. If you are just starting out and your schedule is open, maintaining your website and learning about SEO might be a viable strategy – for the short-term.

But what will happen when your schedule fills up and you no longer have the bandwidth to control your online campaign? Your staff will be busy with their duties. That only leaves one solution: Hire a digital marketing company.

There are many choices out there when it comes to dental marketing firms that specialize in online marketing. As a person dedicated to his or her success – which is likely why you became a dental professional to begin with – you don't want to leave your online success to chance. Nor do you want to find yourself tricked by the false promises and shady marketing tactics other companies may offer.

By the time you are finished reading this book, we are confident that you will find us the ideal digital marketing firm for your long-term success. However, you should realize that hiring a digital marketing company like ours is not a simple transaction.

We are not one of those marketing companies that takes your money and then slinks into the background. In order to get the most out of your digital marketing efforts, you would need to partner with us and follow our proven guidelines.

With our help, you can take control of how your staff operates and interacts with patients daily. You will be able to easily manage the daily processes that govern your office, which in turn will help your staff build better habits over time. As we've seen time and again, this continuous effort and attention will usually lead to a boost in staff morale and an improved patient experience. Best of all, it will bolster your reputation - both online and offline.

Whether you have no web presence at all or you've dabbled in digital marketing before – or you've passed the tasks off to your staff – we can help you create or tighten up your digital marketing efforts so that you can <u>attract the types of patients you prefer</u>.

Not tire kickers, but patients who value excellent dentistry, and who have the insurance or who don't mind paying for skilled service and state-of-the-art dental appliances.

Those patients are what separate the mediocre dental offices with the successful ones, after all. Patients who know the value of implants over dentures, for example, and who maintain a regular dental health routine, including bi-yearly office visits.

That is the beauty of digital marketing. You specify your audience, and you can draw-in those individuals one web page, email or social advertisement at a time.

The qualities of the ideal patient and the details to include in your campaign will be specific to your office, but digital marketing can be customized however you want!

Your goals are only limited by your vision and how hard you're willing to work. We can provide you with the tools. It is up to you how to use them.

First, you may want to know a little more about who we are.

About Firegang Dental Marketing

Firegang Dental Marketing has been helping dental professionals grow their businesses for a decade. During that time we have seen many changes with Google, Facebook, and other online platforms. Despite these alterations, we have managed to build a trustworthy and reliable foundation that is based on *proven* and *consistent* dental marketing strategies for *dependable* results.

Established Company

From the day of our inception, we have worked with hundreds of dental professionals, many who thought they could handle their online dental marketing all on their own. Overwhelmingly, most doctors we work with comment that they should have called us years prior. They then go on to list the amounts of dollars lost, and time wasted, chasing every false promise and shiny object that caught their eye.

Ethical SEO

Digital marketing is ubiquitous and unfortunately infiltrated by more charlatans than we care to admit. These fakers bring down the value of *proven strategy firms* like ours and make otherwise promising dental professionals soured on the entire concept of online marketing.

Our job is to present you with a guide that eases your stress and answers your questions as far as what works, what doesn't, and how best to use your resources as a dental professional.

Expert Marketers

To better assist you, we have gathered together some of the best digital marketing specialists the world over. These individuals are experts at helping dental practices just like yours find new patients online.

Our team's specialty is helping your online presence appeal to the younger generations who grew up with the Internet and who use the web to find local businesses like yours. Because, as you know, capturing this younger audience's attention isn't easy. That's where we come in.

We use only the most advanced techniques that have been proven to work time and again, including advanced Search Engine Optimization (SEO), Google Maps Optimization, Local Search Marketing, Reputation Management, Google AdWords Advertising, Facebook Advertising, and many others.

Proven Tactics

Ours is an efficient system that is based on years of intensive research, and millions spent on rigorous A/B split testing. We have also gathered together the best knowledge, education, and resources from large-scale industry experts around the world. In short, we can confidently say that we know what works and what doesn't, and we are ready to prove it to you.

We have seen glittery objects, and empty promises, come and go, and yet our company has experienced consistent growth while the competition has wavered. When you work with us, you can rest assured that our proprietary system works. While not conventional, it will get you to your end goal, if you follow our process to the letter.

Results Tracking

Building a robust online presence is critical to your success in today's inter-connected world. After all, how will anyone find you when searching Google for dentistry if you have no website? But if you don't track your results, you're not doing your efforts any good. And you might be doing things inefficiently, leading to needless spending and more wasted time.

That is why we make a point to track every result. We're talking web traffic, emails opened, and Facebook ads that resulted in a phone call. Properly tracking your digital campaign's results is so important to digital marketing that it should be one of your top priorities.

Without tracking data, you won't know where your marketing efforts are most paying off, or which ones might not be performing at all. You won't know how best to use your time, energy or money; and that can leave you frustrated and ready to throw in the towel. We have seen it time and again with many offices that neglect proper tracking, which is like trying to find your way in the dark. You'll get somewhere, but you won't know where.

Dedicated Partner

Let us be your guiding light. Here is all you should know about getting your practice noticed online and chosen by quality patients in your area. You can think of this as our initial consultation, in which we would analyze your web presence – if you have one currently – and give you a step-by-step process as to how to strengthen it for mass appeal. Most importantly, we will show you how to maximize your return on investment. That's what digital marketing is all about, after all.

You can use this book in one of several ways. If you're savvy enough, you can use the proven techniques in this book and take the do-it-yourself route. We don't recommend this avenue unless you are experienced with SEO and are able to look at your current business practices with a discerning and subjective eye.

If you are already working with a marketing company, use this advice to determine whether you are getting the most out of your investment. Chances are, you will see that we go further than any other marketing company out there, so there won't be as much overlap between this advice and their work as you might expect. Still, this advice can help you select the best partner for your business, whether it means kicking your current company into shape or hiring a new company to take the digital reigns.

The third way, which is the avenue we suggest, is to partner with us. Firegang will analyze your practice from the bottom up - your online presence, the way your staff answers the phones, and what sets you apart from the rest in town to create a journey for the dental consumer that is irresistible, and that results in maximum return.

Whichever way you choose to use this book, what follows is the best advice you can find on how to build a successful dental practice in the digital age. I wish you all the best. Contact us anytime if you would like to learn more.

To your success,

- Adam Zilko

CHAPTER 1: WHY DIGITAL EXCELLENCE?

When we first sat down to write this book, we wanted to create a resource that stood out while standing the test of time. We started by consuming every digital marketing resource we could find. We scoured bookstores, bought volumes by the dozen on Amazon, and became great friends with our UPS delivery driver. We downloaded free ebooks and whitepapers and spoke with consultants to get a general idea of what information was available, and what new (often empty) promises were being made. Most importantly, we wanted to know the kinds of results dental marketers were getting with the latest and greatest digital marketing tools and tactics used today.

By taking a comprehensive look at the current online marketing landscape as it relates to dentistry, we were able to fulfill our goal. This book, from the very first to its current edition, represents a complete step-by-step guide you can use to take your dental practice to new heights.

How to Use This Book

Become Focused

This book contains three essential parts. The first represents the mental preparation required for getting the most out of this advice. You probably wouldn't expect there to be a "mental edge" side to digital marketing, like you might with boxing, wrestling, or marathon running.

However, just like winning a race or making an opponent submit, you must want it badly enough if you hope to make digital marketing work for you. This point is drastically overlooked in other resources about digital and dental marketing, and yet it's so important to your success.

FIREGANG FACT: If you aren't willing to work hard and put in the hours required to optimize your dental practice, the very best digital marketing campaign in the world will only yield mediocre, if any, results.

Wanting it Badly Enough

You can reap countless rewards from digital marketing. You can fulfill every goal you've established for yourself. But first, you must take action. This is where having the proper mindset is paramount.

Clearing the Negativity

You won't find tips on meditation or positive thinking in this section, though any techniques that put you in the proper headspace couldn't hurt. Instead, we will dispel common myths, correct common mistakes, and put you on the right track mentally to win this game of digital dental marketing.

Building-Out & Fortifying Your Digital Presence

The second part of this book discusses the basics of putting together a fully-customized digital marketing campaign. You will learn the nuts and bolts of how to research and plan a campaign, as well as the basics of search engine optimization, local SEO, and keyword research. Every step presented in these sections is free or low-cost and has the potential to yield amazing results.

Of course, your results will depend on your current market conditions, how well you hold up to your end of the bargain, and how precisely you follow our advice. However, not to worry. We have made every effort to make this information as straightforward as possible so that you spend your time, money, and resources wisely.

Paid Search, Tracking, and Testing

The third part of this book includes the steps required to supercharge your digital marketing campaign. While the first and second parts will help to establish a foundation for your digital presence, the third part helps to build upon your efforts for even greater reach and return.

Paid search marketing and ad retargeting, for example, will put your advertisements in front of prospective new dental patients on Google and Facebook. You will also learn how to track your digital marketing efforts to determine where your work is most paying off and where more attention might be needed.

Finally, you will learn the methods for testing and troubleshooting various elements of your campaign so that you can patch up those cracks that might be bleeding leads or preventing appointments from being scheduled.

By the time you are finished with this book, you will know the basics of how to take a digital campaign from nothing to new heights, for we have created an all-in-one blueprint that all dental marketers can follow to ultimately reach their professional goals (provided your goals are realistic and all other conditions are optimal).

What Kinds of Results Can Expect from Using This Book?

"Results" is such a subjective term. While one dentist may be thrilled with five new patients, another dentist in the same town might only be happy with ten or fifteen. Regardless of which areas you are targeting, what areas you specialize in, what types of new patients you hope to gain, and what your goals happen to be, we can promise you this: If you do the work and put this advice into action, you will gain the following benefits in spades.

Digital Marketing Benefit #1: More New Patients

You don't open your office each morning, fire up your machines and pipe in pleasing music to entertain yourself and your staff. You do it to provide the most memorable experience for your patients. And without the satisfied men, women, teenagers, and children who sit in your chair each day, your office wouldn't remain open for very long.

Our goal is to jampack your schedule from New Year's Day to the end of the holidays, whereby you can continue growing year after year. Once again, what you do with this advice is up to you; but you will have the tools in your possession to reach your objectives in the areas of patient attraction, retention, and return on investment.

Digital Marketing Benefit #2: Improved Income

One of the most popular goals we hear from dental professionals is a desire to earn more. This is not beyond the realm of possibility. With more new patients will undoubtedly come more revenue that can go toward your salary, your staff's salary, and the practice in the form of machine upgrades, add-on renovations, or move to a new location.

Follow these steps and you could be on your way to earning significantly more than you are right now. If that excites you, keep reading. It only gets better from here – as long as you maintain the proper mindset, use the most powerful digital tools and harness the most advanced, tried-and-true dental marketing techniques.

Digital Marketing Benefit #3: Dependable Results

You are busy running your practice and servicing your patients daily. You don't have time to waste on marketing techniques that don't work. The methods you will learn in this book have been thoroughly analyzed, tested to exhaustion, and sharpened by years of trial and error by seasoned marketing professionals. In other words, the methods found on these pages are the most consistent and useful that currently exist. We stake our reputation on it.

First, What Are Your Goals?

Every digital marketing campaign – just like a road map – needs a clear beginning and ultimate end. You already know where you are starting from. Either you have no web presence to speak of, or yours is faltering. You may have a website and a few social profiles, but no paid advertisements. Or, you could have a fully-fledged digital marketing campaign that isn't going anywhere. These elements represent your starting point. They are where you will begin your digital marketing journey.

Your task is to imagine where you want your dental practice to be *three* to *five* years from now. Don't be afraid to dream big. In fact, we encourage it. When setting your campaign goals, it is perfectly okay if you find your head in the clouds; as long as you also keep your feet planted firmly on the ground.

Your "Dream Big" Moment

What do you hope to get out of this journey into dental digital marketing? Do you want to add a thousand more square feet to your current location? Do you want to build a chain of dental offices in every major city? Or quite possibly, you have more modest pursuits.

Whatever you hope to achieve with digital marketing, now is time to make a promise to yourself. This is your chance to let your imagination fly, to stretch your creativity and imagine what life could be like with a bustling office, well-trained staff, and an optimized digital marketing presence that performs like clockwork.

Considered your major, long-term goal, you can make this objective more vivid in your mind by writing it below. Then, be sure to look at it regularly in the coming months to remind yourself why you are harnessing the power of digital marketing in the first place.

I, _____ hope, through digital marketing, to accomplish the following major, long-term goal(s).

_____
_____
_____
_____
_____
_____
_____

Signed: _____
Date: _____

Setting SMART Goals

Using your imagination to dream big is one thing, but it is also important to be realistic. Your goal might be to have a chain of dental offices, but something that monumental isn't going to happen overnight. It is more helpful to set smaller, more achievable goals, which SMART goals are perfect for.

The SMART in SMART Goals stands for:

Specific

This is where you get down to brass tacks. What do you really hope to gain from digital marketing? Think new patients, emergency dentistry cases, or more full-mouth reconstructions. The idea here is to be absolutely concrete about what you expect from your digital marketing campaign.

Measurable

You should be able to identify *when* your goals have been achieved. You can do this by stating that you want a certain amount of Leads, Patients, New Cases, or Dollars Earned. If you want more mouth reconstruction cases, for example, how many will it take for you to feel satisfied?

Achievable

Your goal must be realistic. If you are just starting out and trying to overtake the online presence of a competitor who is already 15-years ahead of the game, and who has been investing thousands of dollars into state-of-the-art digital marketing, you have a huge obstacle to climb. If, on the other hand, you want two new patients this month, or ten new patients this year, those goals are very achievable with the right efforts.

Relevant

The goals you establish for yourself should be relevant to your "Dream Big" goals. For instance, if you hope to build a chain of offices in the next ten years, ten new patients this year will certainly help your current office expand. You might also plan to partner with a marketing company to make expansion more likely to happen.

Time-Bound

How long are you giving yourself to complete your SMART goals? These times should be stated, whether you want more new patients in three months or more dollars earned in five years.

Using the SMART guidelines, come up with one or more milestones you hope to achieve in the coming months and years with the help of digital marketing.

_____
_____
_____
_____
_____
_____
_____
_____

Getting Started

We advise that you approach this book in one of two ways. The first method is to read the book from beginning to end, absorbing and learning the steps as you go. Only then, once you have finished your first read-through, should you go back to the beginning and start putting the steps into action.

However, if you are hungry and anxious to progress, we recommend the other method, which is to start putting these tips into action starting now. The best movers and shakers in this business don't hesitate. They *act* using tried and true methods. We can give you the tools, but you must put them to use if you want them to work.

Whatever you do, don't give up. Only with constant and consistent effort can you hope to achieve your goals, no matter how competitive your market.

CHAPTER 2: GETTING YOUR MIND RIGHT FOR DIGITAL SUCCESS

It is our personal belief that your attitude will determine your success in any industry, and digital marketing is no different. You must be willing to develop the right mindset if you want to make the most impact.

Instead of seeing yourself as a practitioner, you must think like a CEO. Rather than concerning yourself with saving pennies, you should be focusing on generating income by *cutting costs* while *growing your revenue*. Putting a healthy investment into digital marketing is the path to that growth, but you must transition your *mindset* first.

And yet, in our experience, it is incredibly difficult for our clients to alter their customary ways of thinking. And again, doing so is critical to your success. It is your "customary way of thinking" that we encourage you to focus on now.

CEO-minded dentists see marketing companies not as an added expense, but as a tool to be used for goal achievement. CEOs know that success rarely happens in a vacuum and it is only by partnering with like-minded professionals that real growth can occur.

How to Develop A CEO Mindset

Dedicate Yourself to Action

By committing yourself to seeing your actionable steps through to completion, you are adopting the mentality of a business leader. If you remain dedicated to doing your part, you will be well on your way to meeting your goals.

Focus on Progress, Not Perfection

A marketing company is not a fix-all. It's about working as a team to evaluate where you are now versus where you want to be, then making constant improvements until you get there. Focus on making small increases every day. Over time, those minor changes lead to huge results. Focus on getting a little better every day, week, month, and year. And if you make a mistake or fall back a few steps? It won't matter very much. Get back on track and keep on trucking!

Think Long-Term

Leaders of business think long-term whereas employees think short-term. You need to reprogram your mind to think years into the future. Nothing worth accomplishing happens overnight. Therefore, we recommend a long-term commitment to your marketing agency; once you find the right one.

Keep Learning

Never assume that you know everything about marketing your dental practice online. You must be a student of your business and how it interacts with prospects and patients in the digital age. Educate yourself on the buyer cycle, conversion funnel, proper phone answering techniques, and how to maximize every opportunity.

Embrace Risk Taking

Business and marketing, at their core, are about taking risks. That doesn't mean you should gamble your kid's college fund on red at the local casino. Instead, we are referring to the more calculated risks that allow you to determine what's working and what's not. That knowledge will then let you change what's not working so you can continuously advance.

It is far riskier to do little or nothing at all.

Pledge yourself to take risks and realize that developing and tailoring a marketing plan to best suit your needs begins with a calculated risk that is then tweaked to precision.

Have Realistic Expectations and Timelines

We spoke about expectations and timelines a moment ago when you devised your SMART goals. We are revisiting those ideas here because it is important for you to be realistic when hiring a marketing agency.

We would be overjoyed if we could make a massive impact on your business in a short period of time. Unfortunately, marketing is a long-term affair, and it may be months or years before you begin to see the juiciest fruits of your marketing efforts.

Without realistic expectations, you may start to feel burned or cheated as your campaign progresses. And meanwhile, your agency will begin to feel powerless. Instead, it is critical that you both agree on what is achievable in the agreed-upon timeframe and within the budget you have available.

Invest in Your Business

Many dentists tend to hold back when it comes to marketing, either on the decision to hire a company or to invest sufficiently in that company once the agreement is signed. This "wait and see" approach can be detrimental to your practice and goals.

However, we are going to go a step further. The hesitancy to invest money, while understandable, will ultimately harm your business. Period. You may have very achievable goals, but if you aren't willing to invest the time and money it takes to reach those goals, then you're just biding your time until a new dentist, big corporation, or multi-location dentist opens its doors nearby, vying for the same patients.

Unfortunately, by then it will take a much more significant investment to compete. Invest now to prevent your competitors from attaining the upper hand.

Do the Work

Wait, you may be thinking, there's work involved?

Ideally, you would establish your goals, and your marketing company would take those goals and make them a reality. Unfortunately, the company you partner with cannot do all of the work for you.

Just like your patients can't rely solely on your expertise to keep their teeth clean and healthy (they must do their part twice per day, every day, after all), you must be willing to train your staff, monitor their calls, and keep everyone motivated so that every milestone is reached.

Do you have the proper CEO mindset? We hope so. Working with a marketing agency offers many benefits, from shortening the learning curve to getting faster results. We can provide you with the necessary skills and training, hold you accountable, and motivate you to succeed. But without the mentality of a business leader, you won't get half as far.

Starting with a Clean Slate – Dispelling Common Digital Marketing Myths

Have you ever heard "misinformation" disguised as "facts" when it comes to digital marketing? How would you know? We can help.

For this advice to work, you will need to get rid of all preconceived notions so that you can start fresh, without any adverse perceptions or incorrect advice hindering your results.

By dispelling the following myths, we can eliminate any confusion that can cause significant problems later. We want you to be on the same page so that you may reap the most benefits from your marketing efforts.

Myth #1: Word-of-mouth referrals are better than any form of marketing, including digital.

The Truth

Many doctors call us, even though they are still skeptical. They simply fail to see how digital marketing can make any sort of ripple in their patient numbers.

We do concede that word-of-mouth is of the utmost importance, with 92% of consumers stating that they would trust a word-of-mouth recommendation from a friend or relative. But this doesn't have to be an either/or debate.

Word-of-mouth is necessary, that much is certain, but mentioning a good dentist to a friend is not a stand-alone experience. Most will venture straight to Google to learn more about the doctor in question. They will look at the listing to see how high it shows up on Google's Search Engine Results Page (SERP). They will judge the color scheme and graphics of the doctor's website. They will read the most recent online reviews and – in an instant – decide if the recommendation they just received from their friend or co-worker is legit (or not).

In other words, whether it's word-of-mouth, a sandwich board on the street corner or a flyer in the mail, there is no single new patient scenario today that does not involve *at least* one touchpoint with your digital presence.

Therefore, instead of thinking of digital marketing as a new marketing method that costs an exorbitant amount of time and money, think of it as a necessary supplement to the marketing techniques you currently have in place. That includes the word-of-mouth referrals you receive due to the reputation you have worked so hard to establish in your local community.

Relying solely on referrals is not the way to go. Waiting for referrals to call or walk-in is a passive exercise, and one that sets yourself up for failure. You are relying on chance and betting your future on the whims of the universe. You might as well base your digital marketing on tea leaf readings or the ramblings of a Ouija board.

In other words, instead of focusing solely on referrals to keep patients in your chair, be active and strive to be wherever your patients are likely to make contact with your online presence. The bottom line is that word-of-mouth referrals can help, but digital marketing can accelerate the results from that and all other offline lead generation efforts.

Myth #2: Established practices will always have the upper hand.

The Truth

It used to take decades for a dental practice to establish a trustworthy reputation in the local community. Digital marketing has changed that. Now, instead of taking years to get prospects' attention, even newly-opened practices can make a splash in a short amount of time.

With the help of advanced digital marketing tools and strategies, you can reach out to your patients wherever they happen to be. They could be at work on their desktops or out and about on their smartphones. They could even be parked in front of the TV on their tablets. With digital marketing, you can speak to these individuals on their level, even the younger, more tech-savvy generations, and you can remain fresh on the minds of prospective patients without being pushy or intrusive.

Digital marketing is key if you hope to dominate your local market, and we will show you how to do just that. Whether yours is the newest practice in town or a community staple, we have the answers you desire for growth.

Myth #3: Digital marketing can yield instant results.

The Truth

While quick results are possible - such as five or ten new patients in a month - expanding to a new practice in a month is unlikely. Unfortunately, there exist more than a few digital marketing charlatans who offer "too good to be true" results. They may advertise: "Sign up now, and you can earn 2000 new leads in a single month!" Or they may assure you that you can sign up 100 new patients this year! The fact is, no one can guarantee those kinds of results, and if you are ever promised instant or even rapid digital marketing results like these – run away and don't look back.

While it is true that some clients get lucky and experience quick-burst results right out of the gate, most forms of digital marketing take time before measurable advancements become apparent.

Your rate of success depends on your location and current market conditions. It relies on the state of your online presence and how quickly you acclimate to the constantly-evolving digital landscape while being consistent with the most advanced marketing techniques.

We can promise you this. The sooner you act, the quicker you will be able to take control of your online reputation, and the faster you can start making things happen for your dental practice.

Myth #4: I can hire a marketing company and then set and forget.

The Truth

Many of the doctors and staff we work with are overwhelmed at our insistence that we don't just take their money and then slink quietly away into the background.

That is because so many dental practices have been taken for granted in the past, and an unfortunately high number of doctors have been burned. Many have hired SEO companies in the past, some to the tune of thousands of dollars per month, only now they have nothing at all to show for it.

These SEO companies sent out a report every now and again to show they were working, but the results the doctors expected never came.

From the beginning, we have been driven to be different. As digital marketing professionals, our clients know us for our willingness and ability to dig in deep and get into the trenches with your dentistry staff.

With years of experience behind us, we analyze how your front desk staff is answering the phones, and if leads are being called back quickly and with a caretaker's approach.

We look for weaknesses in scheduling to ensure patients are keeping to their appointments. At the same time, we build out your online presence so that prospects looking for a new dental professional in town see your listing on their computers, smartphones, or tablets.

In summary, your success is dependent upon your active engagement with us. We are not a set-and-forget organization. You must do some of the work.

It's like this: What if you had a patient sit in your chair and ask you to give them a healthy and beautiful smile, but they didn't want to engage in any oral hygiene practices at home? They didn't want to brush or floss or rinse. Instead, they merely wanted to visit you twice a year; and for that, they wanted to be able to enjoy a perfect smile.

What would you say to that patient?

Impossible, right? Digital Marketing is no different. You must do some of the work to yield maximum results.

Myth #5: A small digital marketing budget goes a long way.

The Truth

Investing *more* is often the hardest pill to swallow for new clients. You cannot hope to expand from one practice to three in a year, and in a highly-competitive market, without a substantial digital marketing budget.

On the other hand, you might be able to get away with a minimal budget to dominate your local market if yours is one of only two dental offices in town.

Here's a better way to look at it: Your financial investment must be proportional to the goals you hope to achieve, the level of aggressiveness you wish to put forth in attaining those goals, and the obstacles you face along the way.

There is no such thing as a free lunch, in nature, business, dentistry, or digital marketing.

Here's another way to consider the amount you should allow for your digital marketing budget: What do you tell your patients who may be considering cheaper dental implants or going to an unskilled doctor for a less expensive root canal? You would highly advise against it, not only because you want the business and revenue, but because you care about the safety and oral health of your patients! You don't want to send them to a bargain-bin alternative, because – as with most things – you truly do get what you pay for.

Does digital marketing have to cripple you financially? Of course not. Just keep in mind that a bigger budget is sometimes necessary if you hope to overtake all obstacles in a highly-competitive market. The only caveat is that you must know what you are doing.

Free techniques can yield results, but the right amount of capital focused in the right directions can yield 8 to 10 times greater results for your dental practice.

The trick is to plan your marketing investment properly so that you achieve a healthy return.

Myth #6: All you need to succeed at digital marketing is a website.

The Truth

You could have the biggest, baddest website in your local area with flashing lights, photos of picture-perfect teeth, and all the bells and whistles needed to attract quality patients. However, if your super-duper website doesn't succeed at converting visitors into actual patients, what do you even have it for?

Most digital marketing foundations start with a website, as that is where most prospective new patients will venture to learn more about you. And that is precisely what you want. The alternative is to have a third party like DentalTown inform prospects of your background and services, and who knows what kind of information they will convey. Do you really want to take that chance?

Your website is like your home base, but it is only one small aspect of a fully-functional digital marketing campaign.

Correcting Common Digital Marketing Mistakes

Now that we have dispelled those infectious and dangerous myths – dangerous because they threaten your time, money, and reputation – it is time to discuss the blunders we have seen dental marketers commit many times over.

Even if you are not committing any of the mistakes below, you should still know about them. That way, you can refrain from making any of them in the future. You will be tempted, especially when it comes to the first point, as everyone seems to want to veer off track right soon after getting started. But we assure you, if you avoid these mistakes, you will grease the skids to achieving your major and SMART goals.

Mistake #1: Chasing every false promise and shiny object.

Imagine if, after examining a patient, you took the time to plan a detailed dental treatment plan, only for the patient to want to diverge from that plan months or years into the process? It would frustrate you, wouldn't it? You are the dental expert, after all. Why isn't the patient listening to your professional opinion and guidance?

This experience is akin to the way digital marketing clients want to switch months or years into their campaigns, mostly because they are not seeing the results they expected.

FIREGANG FACT: It can take 24 to 36 months for your website to be truly optimized, though many of our clients see significant results much sooner than that.

Dental professionals, marketers, and consultants alike are all guilty of jumping from one technique to the next in the hopes that one will produce immediate and substantial results. There are no quick fixes and jumping from method to method will only force you to go right back to where you started—at the beginning—instead of allowing gradual results to produce substantial changes down the line.

We recommend that you follow our advice and stay the course if you hope for long-term and lasting results.

Mistake #2: Not having a dedicated digital marketing budget.

We get it. You want to grow your dental practice, and you want to do it for as little money as possible. A mindset like that is destined for success, and that's a very good thing.

But here is something else to consider: You will not reach your SMART or "Dream Big" goals without dedicating a certain amount to marketing each month. Your practice may need to spend $2000-$4000 per month, or you may only need to maintain a modest budget of $500. Your marketing expenditure will depend on your area, market, the state of your online presence, as well as your reputation within the local community.

The amount you should allocate to digital marketing will also depend on the strength of your competition and the aggressiveness of any moves they may have made in the digital landscape.

And as we've said, your budget will depend on how aggressively you wish to achieve your goals, and how quickly.

FIREGANG FACT: To remain competitive, a digital marketing budget should be maintained that is congruent with your practice goals. Most practices would do well with a 5%-7% investment. The exception is a client in a hypercompetitive market or a new startup looking to make a splash quickly in a saturated field.

There is no "one size fits all" answer to how much money your practice should spend on marketing. Someone starting out may need to invest *more* while someone in a smaller market may need *less* to make an impact.

But the fact remains, you need a marketing budget in place, and much of it should be focused on digital, as that's where your prospects are likely to be.

Mistake #3: Delaying decisions until it's too late.

Don't let this book be another one that you flip through and promptly set down, never to think of it again. The world is always advancing, which means that the longer you delay marketing your practice online, the harder it will be to get in front of interested prospects when you finally do act.

The big-name practices and chains in the industry are successful because they make bold moves quickly without an ounce of hesitation. Whether it's putting together an innovative marketing blitz or a series of expensive TV commercials, these star players know that those who hesitate usually *stagnate*.

These movers and shakers may not always return dividends, but they learn from their mistakes and use the data they glean to make their next moves even more powerful.

This is the mindset to adopt if you hope to compete with the dental giants among you.

Mistake #4: Treating leads as an afterthought

The entire purpose of digital marketing is to get prospective patients into your chair. It's the same motivation you have when putting up a billboard, securing a TV spot or placing an ad in the local newspaper: You want more eyeballs, attention, and business.

Therefore, you should expect for the phone to start ringing and your lobby to be bustling once your digital campaign is optimized. While that won't happen overnight, it will happen eventually. It's what you then do with those inbound leads that makes all the difference.

When a person sees your website in the Google search results, and then clicks-through, they are deciding that you may be better than all the rest. They are still in the research phase - or the discovery phase - of the buyer's journey, which we will discuss in a later chapter.

For now, put yourself in a web visitor's shoes. They land on your website, read enough content, and see enough visual appeal to call your office phone number.

Now, what if this prospective new patient called your office only to be treated with indifference? Or what if they called only to be put on hold for several minutes?

What if someone calls your office after-hours? Do you have an answering staff that is prepared to log the required information so that lead can be called back later? Most importantly, are all leads being called back in a timely manner and with as much caring enthusiasm as your staff can muster?

Because, to be frank, your staff should be calling back leads without delay to answer questions, make prospects feel comfortable, and help them schedule an appointment.

If that's not happening, no amount of marketing or advertising will help you succeed, digital or otherwise.

Mistake #5: Trying to do everything yourself or not delegating properly.

Many clients come to us after they have attempted to create or retool their website or social profiles, or they have delegated tasks to their staff with disastrous results.

The Wrong Way to Delegate Responsibility

Want to hear a horror story? We had one client who had been working with us for years. With both an organic SEO and paid search campaign running side-by-side, we had achieved lead generation and lead conversion numbers we were all happy with. The client was satisfied, and so were we. The digital campaign we had devised for the good doctor was on track for greatness, full steam ahead.

This particular dental practice employed an office manager who was quite ambitious. In thinking that she could save the doctor money, she told our client about the savings she had discovered.

Our client, not really understanding what savings she was referring to, gave her the go-ahead to put her plan into action. What could it hurt, he thought? After all, every bit of revenue saved does the practice an ounce of good.

When we visited the client's office the next day, we discovered that the website we had constructed for the doctor was down. All of the links pointing to the website from paid advertisements and other online methods were broken, which meant that all the efforts we had put into place for the past several years had been decimated in one fell swoop.

Unbeknownst to us or the doctor, the office manager received a call from a competing marketing company and thought she could save her boss thousands by switching to their organization in the middle of our digital campaign.

It was very much like fitting a patient with braces only for that patient to go to a competitor to have your appliances removed in place of his "shiny new" braces.

Even though we were able to get the campaign back online a short time later, the damage had been done. It then took even more time to return the campaign back to where we had it after years of diligent work.

The point is, only by staying the course and delegating responsibly can you hope to achieve your goals. There are some things that can be done by your staff, like answering emails that come in from your website, and answering the phones in a friendly and helpful manner.

However, when it comes to optimizing your website, tweaking your paid ads, analyzing your Internet traffic data, and testing and improving your campaigns, some things are simply better left to the experts.

To delegate responsibly, pay attention to the individual skills and talents of your staff members. Stacy, who possesses the stellar social skills, might be better on the phones while Pat, who is better at organization, might be better suited for scheduling. Social media-savvy staff members can handle the social posting, and you can divvy up other responsibilities as necessary to keep your digital marketing efforts progressing as you expect.

Mistake #6: Not knowing how to identify the experts

Whether you run your office in Houston or Phoenix, Memphis or Jacksonville, you are likely inundated with calls from SEOs and marketing companies alike. It can become tedious sorting through all those calls, wondering who to trust and wishing for a simpler solution.

When you get solicited by a marketing company, or even if you have sought the company out, the interaction typically begins with the SEO rep asking if you are happy with your marketing. Or they may even mention Google marketing specifically.

If you have ever worked with any of these companies or entertained next steps, you know that they all charge different amounts and employ a variety of tools and processes. But once you hire those companies, how can you be sure that any work is being done? On one hand you have companies that send the occasional "update" email filled with gobbledygook you hardly understand, and then there are the companies that send a report every month - but, again, who can decipher them?

The worst companies become entirely unresponsive the moment you sign on the dotted line. Funny how your check always gets cashed though, isn't it?

Sadly, there are too many charlatans in the digital marketing industry. The Internet is still very much a Wild, Wild, West, and snake oil salespeople still abound. Legal resource [HG.org](HG.org) went as far as to ask, "Is the SEO Industry 80% Scam?"

Certainly scams exist, in SEO and in nearly every other industry. Credit card companies and even designer purse manufacturers have to worry about fraud, too. However, as a dental professional, you should be able to discern between the worthy and worthless. You should know when to say, "Yes, let's do business!" and when you should turn on your heels and walk away.

After all, if you are going to toil away at anything as monumental as digital marketing, you may as well do it right; and with a properly trained, experienced and motivated team guiding your way.

The problem is that it is often difficult to know when you are working with someone legitimate and when someone may be doing very little when you expect so much.

Do your research, trust your gut, and choose the company that fills you with the most inspiration to achieve your desired goals.

Ready to Get Started?

Now that you are thinking like a dental CEO, have no misconceptions and can avoid the common mistakes many clients make, you are ready to plan your digital marketing campaign. Or, as we like to call it, your "Digital Marketing Treatment Plan."

CHAPTER 3: CREATING YOUR DIGITAL MARKETING "TREATMENT PLAN"

Just as you wouldn't begin a patient's root canal or fit a patient with Invisalign without a detailed plan, so it goes with digital marketing.

And, as with any dental plan, a proper analysis should be conducted. This thorough examination will include your local market and demographics information. For instance, you should know where your prospects live, including the towns, cities, suburbs, and counties, how much they earn per year, and what they want in a dental professional.

Only then can you hope to create a plan that will yield steady and long-lasting results. However, a plan is definitely needed. You wouldn't just set a ship in the water and hope that it reaches its destination. Especially when your competition has an armada decked out with the latest tech and a course set dead-ahead.

No, to compete in today's rapidly-paced market, you need the very best tools, technologies, and guidance by your side.

FIREGANG FACT: There is no "one size fits all" to digital marketing, but you must start with best-practices as your foundation, then test and test again to discover what your audience best responds to.

The challenge with creating a book like this is that there is no cookie-cutter way to make digital marketing work for you. We mention this for several reasons.

Market Conditions Vary

Going into a competitive market like Miami, Florida, is going to require much more diligent work, a long-term commitment, and an extensive marketing budget as opposed to a smaller, less-competitive market like Lake Charles, Louisiana.

A cookie-cutter plan simply couldn't account for these market variations, and anyone who tells you differently is leading you blindly into uncertain territory. Spend your marketing budget wisely.

Dental Offices are Unique

No dental practice is the same. You might have one that accepts Medicaid and one that only accepts Blue Cross Blue Shield. The marketing approaches to capture the attention and information of these audiences is going to depend on several factors.

The point is, you can't just slap a digital marketing plan into place and expect to get a return. Few things in life work that way. However, we have succeeded in creating a digital marketing "foundation" that you can customize to make your own and then expand upon.

It's like tooth bonding. You can use it to fill cracks and carries, or you can create full mouth reconstructions. Whatever your goals happen to be, our system can be molded to get you there.

Treatment Plan Step 1: Aligning with Your End Goal

Your digital marketing treatment plan, as we like to call it, is where you turn back to your major and SMART goals. You must know what you want to accomplish, when, and how.

During this stage, you must also identify the radius of your target market. We recommend seven miles to most clients, but your area could be different. You could live in a rural market where the closest neighbors are 20 minutes away. You should be able to identify the local areas you hope to target by name, including all applicable cities, towns, suburbs, and counties, and you should have a record of your area's demographics information, including income levels.

Who Are You Marketing to? Identifying Your Target Market

Geographic Location

Start out by making a list of your geographical area and all terms that would be used to describe it. For example, your list might include the state Texas, the city Houston, the county Harris, as well as the area known as Pasadena to help new patients find you. Your list might be long if you live in a densely populated metropolitan area, or it could be short if you live in a rural area.

Pinpointing the Ideal Patient

FIREGANG FACT: Most local areas have a dedicated Facebook page, where you can find fans and followers to get an idea of *who* you should be marketing to.

Do you have an ideal patient in mind? In marketing speak, this is referred to as a Buyer Persona. Much like a character that you create in a video game, the persona you create will be based on a mix of real-life people. It's an amalgam, if you will, of all the prospective patients in your area.

Create a profile of this patient now. Include demographics information, such as income level, educational background, employment, and other factors that are important to your practice's goals.

By the time you have completed the profile, you should know your ideal patient's income level, hobbies, buying habits and - most importantly - oral care habits. You should also have an idea of how often that person tends to visit the dentist (or require oral surgery or need braces).

Search online for a dentist like a patient

One way to build-out your digital marketing plan is to begin an online search as if you yourself were searching for services just like yours. You might go to Google and type "Dentist in [your town]" or "Orthodontist in Maine," for example.

After hitting submit, spend a few moments analyzing the website listings that populate the first page. Is your website among them? If so, how does your listing appear? Does it stand out? Or is like a drop of water in a sea of blue?

FIREGANG FACT: Google has a vested interest in showing you the results *you* want to see. If you are signed into your Gmail account, the sites you have most visited will show up more prominently in the search results. Searching using an Incognito tab or clearing your

browser cache before searching will give you more accurate organic results. Now, you are searching Google as a prospect who has never visited your website before.

If your site fails to show up on the first page of Google at all, keep clicking through the pages until you find your listing. Then, whether your site is on the first or tenth page, click-through to your website from Google to see what type of site you are greeted with.

Are the colors of your website appealing? Is the information you seek easy to find? Most importantly, do you have one or more ways to ask a question or schedule an appointment right at your fingertips?

An expert will be able to take this journey through your online presence to discover where walls need to be patched up and where new structures need to be built.

If you hired an unskilled SEO company in the past, their efforts may have significantly impaired your rankings, all the way to present day. An experienced eye can discern shoddy SEO work and can help you enact a plan to get you back on track.

No matter what your online presence looks like now, a sleek and advanced digital marketing "Treatment Plan" can put your dental practice in front of prospective patients. How long it takes depends on you, your area, your staff, and how well you follow these steps.

Our goal is to bolster and make prominent your online listings so that you get more clicks to your website. We will also ensure that information is easy to find for all prospects, leading to more emails, phone calls, and visits to your office.

Treatment Plan Step 2: Identifying Your Uniqueness

Never forget that you are offering a valuable service to your patients. It sounds like common sense, but it is incredibly easy to lose sight of this fact when it comes to marketing your practice.

You may find yourself getting so caught up in clicks and visitors and conversion rates that you forget that it's more importantly about your chair-side manner and skilled hands, how well your staff treats new leads and current patients. It's about how clean and orderly your office is, and how satisfied your patients are when they leave your office following their appointments.

All of those elements are common to every dental practice, but you should also never forget that your practice is unique. It is that one-of-a-kind factor that should drive the creation of your digital campaign from start to finish.

A professional digital marketing plan takes into account your office culture, staff personalities, and everyone's skill set and natural abilities, and any digital marketing processes you may already have in place. It also requires you to list if you have any specializations or whether you are a general or cosmetic dentist, for example.

There is no single "right way" to market a dental practice. We have had success putting 100% of our efforts into 24-hour dentistry for one client, and the efforts paid off. We only took that chance after much consideration, research, and the experience we have to fall back on.

You may create "Same Day Crowns" better than another dentist. If so, this should be a campaign priority and mentioned as often as possible to patients who are good candidates for that service.

Or perhaps you want to focus on simple patient acquisition and then do your up-selling while the patient is in the chair, such as offering a new-patient special for only $39!

Then again, marketing your high-end services like Invisalign and implants or veneers and full-mouth reconstructions might interest you more. All of these details should be considered when planning your campaign and with an open and ongoing dialog between dentist and marketing firm.

An effective campaign chooses colors that invoke comfort and familiarity and uses language that is helpful and positive. A good campaign makes prospective patients feel at ease while also showcasing your expertise. It presents you as the best dental professional in town; not right away, but eventually and over time.

If you already have a website, some social media activity, and you have an email newsletter that goes out each month, you are ahead of most practices we work with, but that isn't near enough. For one, is your website optimized? If not, what needs to be changed? Do your emails have subject lines that prospects and patients can't resist? Or are they bland and boring, becoming lost altogether amid the inbox noise?

When devising your treatment plan and the processes it utilizes, you are once again encouraged to dream big. Do you want to change up your colors or your overall image? Now is the time to do so, as once something is on the Internet, it is difficult to remove.

Do you want to offer new services or highlight some services that patients don't ask about, but that deliver more revenue? These are ideas that should all go into your new digital marketing plan.

What Are You Marketing? Analyzing Your Practice

The Strengths of Your Office and Staff

Now is the time to create a list of your practice strengths. Write down the services your practice offers, your office hours, pricing, and the overall message you hope to convey.

While you're at it, take a good look at your staff and make a list of their personal strengths, then try to identify any attributes that can be utilized or improved upon as your campaign progresses. Ongoing training, after all, should always be part of any solid plan.

Treatment Plan Step 3: Eyeing the Competition

It is unlikely that you are the only tooth doctor in town. You probably have at least one and maybe even several more dental professionals vying for the same target audience.

You will soon learn how to identify all of your digital marketing competitors - at least the ones you should be concerned about - to make sense of the Google SERPs.

Using this skill set, you will be able to pinpoint where your competitors are succeeding and where they're falling short. By understanding the opposition, you will be in a far better position to make a dent or even dominate your local area once your campaign is optimized.

It's a fact that patients today have more choices and easier access to dentistry than ever before, barring income and insurance. You have mom-and-pop dental offices that have been passed down through generations and corporate dentists to contend with, and every level of office in between. How can you hope to compete? With digital marketing, that's how.

When patients are no longer limited by choice, their selection depends on the services you offer and how attractive your listings are compared to the other guys to their searching eye.

There are other factors to consider, of course. Online reviews, your reputation in town, your patient track record - these can all affect the results of your digital marketing campaigns - but your listings should be top-notch if you hope to stack the digital deck in your favor.

To get an idea of what it takes to beat-out the competition, conduct a Google search for a dental professional like you in your area. Which of your competitors shows up first?

Whoever it is, do they have lots of five-star reviews while you have few? Make note of these differences, because now you have some objectives to target - either higher rankings, more reviews, gold stars or all of the above.

Also, consider what services and level of service the other dental professionals offer. Can you take advantage of any specials? If you are offering a new-patient special of $120 and your competitor down the street charges $39, you might still get undercut by that dental practice; even if your digital marketing campaign is optimized and on-point.

By thoroughly researching competitors, you won't be taken by surprise by any offers that may steal attention or patients from your office.

Finally, call your competitors and ask them about their digital marketing campaigns and overall efforts. For instance, you can ask about the platforms they use. What areas do they tend to focus on most, and what budgets are they working with?

If you have the gumption to conduct this type of recon work, it can be highly effective at helping you develop a marketing plan that is ultra-competitive.

In our experience, no one knows the competition quite like you do. You are probably very familiar with most, if not all, dental professionals in your immediate area. You probably know the services they offer, and what sets them apart. If not, you should know this information if you want to fortify your digital marketing campaign.

If you were a new client of ours, we would require your input about your competitors at this stage. We would ask you to give us a rundown of all of your competitors and what they seem to be doing better than you. This may not even be factual information. What's most important is your perception of these doctors and how prospects in your area perceive them. That's information we can then use to bolster your campaign.

Organizing Your Data

Keep this location, demographics, and competitor data handy. You will be referring to the information frequently as your dental Internet marketing campaign develops and progresses.

Handwritten lists are great, but it is a far better idea to create a spreadsheet that you can organize, access, search, and filter for easier recall.

The Bare Bones of a Digital Marketing Plan

The information above was designed to help you gather all the details necessary to build-out your digital marketing campaign. It should be noted that, in some cases, you won't get the details exactly right, and some details you may miss altogether.

It is okay to make educated guesses on colors and language used and subject lines written, if you test those details once your campaign has been enacted. Testing, after all, is what separates the unskilled from those digital marketing companies that are worthy of your time and budget.

Once the foundation is created, it's proper testing that helps a campaign become more sharpened and effective over time. But you must know your area and market and competition thoroughly so that you know what to test, and when.

Because, as you may have noticed by now, what works for one dental practice may not work for yours. Similarly, what fell flat for a dentist in Austin or New York may work swimmingly for your office. This is where testing is paramount and should be handled by experts. Testing does little good if you don't know how to test, when, or how to decipher the results to refine your efforts over time.

You may also notice that we keep telling you that you need experts to guide you. That is for a good reason. We have seen far too many practices choose lower-cost SEO companies only to experience the same depressing results. Don't let that happen to you.

The following isn't so much to help you plan a marketing campaign on your own, as it provides a framework to teach you the ropes so that you aren't taken for a ride by an unscrupulous SEO company in the future.

We are educating you so that you can tell the digital marketing experts from those who just started a year ago. You will also be able to take more control over your campaigns and make suggestions using the standards and best-practices listed in this book. Information like this will allow you to step into your market on the right foot.

It won't be easy.

Digital marketing requires a mixture of caution and aggression. You or the marketing company pulling the strings in the background need to be able to make meaningful decisions at a moment's notice, *and* when the time is right. Sometimes this requires you to spend more of your marketing budget, which is an idea that is resisted by many clients at first. But we stress to you that these decisions are never made lightly and could mean the difference between a number one spot in Google and a listing that falls perilously low to page 3.

Right now, you are probably chomping at the bit, ready to learn these easy-to-implement steps that will help your practice reach its true potential. Before we get started, we urge you to look around your office right now. You might even want to take a few pictures. Because things should be a whole lot better a year or even three years from now. And in five years? Who knows where you might be? Look at your major and SMART goals lists to get some ideas.

How to Compete Against Corporate Dental Practices and Win

It is no secret that corporate dental practices are growing. Just take a look at your local community. How many miles away are you from the nearest corporate office? Probably not that far. While this growth in corporate dentistry can certainly be intimidating, it doesn't have to be. It is still possible for small dental offices to fight and win against large competitive forces. The key is to start by understanding corporate strengths and weaknesses. Then, use this information to create a strategy that takes advantage of those weaknesses.

For example, it is extremely difficult for corporate practices to create any sort of personalized experience for the patient. Their websites all look exactly the same regardless of office location, with little to no information about the doctors or staff.

Furthermore, these clone offices typically possess online reviews that are more lackluster than anything, which should offer proof to local prospects that they're not the best choice in town. What's more, these corporate dental practices are simply far too big for their own good. For example, good luck implementing a single marketing change across multiple offices. A move like that would be a headache for the corporates, while your small office may thrive with such a rapid and unexpected maneuver.

By knowing your opposition's weaknesses, you will be in a better position to capitalize on those flaws using the best digital marketing strategies. Let's look at an example.

The team at Timber Dental didn't let corporate offices get them down. They created a personal brand that does everything the corporates can't: Deliver an inviting and personalized experience.

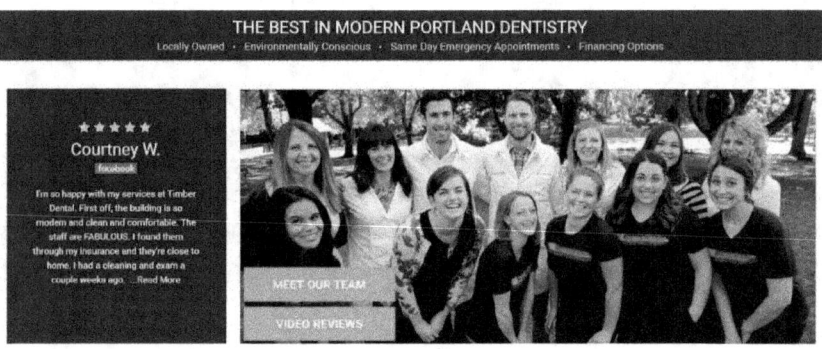

Create a Memorable Online Brand

Digital marketing is all about trust. Anyone can slap a website online, but it's the websites that are trusted that get the most business.

The more trust you can build with potential new patients, the more you can differentiate your dental practice against the corporate offices. Start by creating a memorable brand with your website.

Ensure that your site answers all your new patients' questions. Corporate practices don't have the room to create an educational experience on their websites, but that is exactly what patients want to see.

An About Us page is an excellent way educate and endear your office and staff to prospects and patients. Your About page should be populated with a story about your humble beginnings, your struggles to get where you are today, an explanation of the services you offer, what insurances you accept, and what financing options are available. It should include your mission statement and – above all – what makes your office unique.

The rest of your site should be filled with relevant and high-quality information that is researched, positive, and easily accessible.

The Power of Online Reviews

You can't tell prospects that your office is better and expect to be believed. Instead, you must prove your worth as a dental professional. The way to prove yourself is with Google reviews.

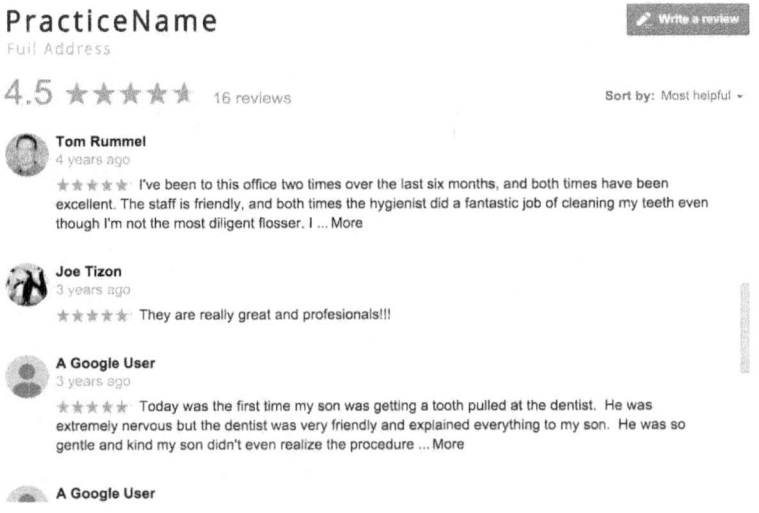

How many Google Reviews does your practice have? What is your overall rating? How do your reviews and rating compare to your competitors operating in the same space?

If prospective patients see that your practice sports an average five-star rating compared to a corporate practice with mostly three-star reviews, which office do you think patients will click on first? Yours, of course.

In this manner, digital marketing – and Google reviews – have effectively leveled the playing field.

The fact is, Google reviews are only going to increase in importance as time goes on. Therefore, ensure that you have an active strategy in place that encourages patients to leave reviews about your practice online. That way, new prospects will be enticed to click on your Google listings over all the other dental offices in town.

CHAPTER 4: MAKE CONVERSIONS YOUR FOCUS

"How will I know when my marketing campaign is optimized?" one of our newest clients recently asked.

Our answer was simple: When there are more new patients in your dental chair.

While that seems the most obvious answer, you can't really blame the client for asking such a basic and necessary question. It is very easy to get distracted in this business. With digital marketing, there are many things to keep track of. There are pages and leads, clicks and phone calls, bounce rates and conversions. So, what's really important?

One of our digital marketing competitors offers new clients a thousand new leads every month. And if the company doesn't come through, the client doesn't have to pay a thing!

Sounds like an excellent offer, doesn't it? Turns out, several of our current clients have tried this too-good-to-be-true offer prior to working with us. Are you anxious to learn the result?

As you might expect, not one of them received a single viable lead to their businesses. Oh, sure, they received a thousand "leads" a month, but these phone calls were from telemarketers and insurance companies and wrong numbers. Should those be considered leads? Our clients didn't think so.

The entire point of digital marketing is to "convert" a prospect into a patient. In other words, "conversions" should always be your focus.

Now, here is where the terminology gets tricky. The overall goal is to attract new patients and earn a higher return, this much is true. However, a conversion can refer to any enticed action online. For instance, a prospect filling out a form on your website is considered a conversion. As is a phone call that comes into your answering service by a prospect who landed on your website.

Even though these prospects are still considered "Leads," they converted, and thus are one step closer to become actual patients.

There are so many numbers and figures to keep track of in digital marketing. But by only focusing on the actions taken - or the conversions - we can more accurately predict what will work in your market.

With our proven system, if your office is getting phone calls and those calls are not being closed, swift action needs to be taken. Those are wasted opportunities, after all. With conversions as your focus, you will soon be able to pinpoint the broken element(s) of your campaign with precision accuracy. That can lead to more closed appointments and the higher ROI on your marketing investment that you expect.

New Patient Buying Cycle

An excellent way to increase your profits is to identify and capitalize on all available opportunities. Anyone calling, emailing or visiting your office is interested in what you offer. You should be trying to close those leads that instant. If you don't or can't, you may lose that prospect forever.

As a dental professional, you need to get into the minds of your prospects and patients. Learn how they think and act, and ultimately how they make their buying decisions.

For instance, what makes a patient choose one dentist over another? What steps do they take before deciding to pick up the phone and call? By understanding how a prospect makes a positive decision, you can alter your marketing campaign to cater to their exact needs.

Just make sure you don't neglect your current patients. Growing your dental practice doesn't just mean acquiring new business. You must also treat, satisfy, and retain the patients you already have.

Identifying your current patients' buying cycle will ultimately help you boost your profits. By knowing how your past and current patients behaved, you can more accurately predict the actions of prospects and new patients.

Every day you and your staff are presented with chances for opportunity. If you're not optimizing every stage of your buying cycle, you are missing out on those critical circumstances that can elevate your practice to the next level.

Farewell to Linear Marketing

A patient's buying process is rarely linear. That is, few will see an ad and call your office right away to book an appointment. There are several steps in between their first and last interaction with your brand that can shape their perception of your practice.

Patients tend to go on a decision-making journey before finally selecting a dental office. By breaking this journey down and understanding it, you will begin to realize the value of each marketing channel and the ROI associated with each stage.

5 Stages of the New Patient Buying Cycle

Stage 1: Problem Recognition

This is the stage when a person begins looking for a dental professional. They may have bitten into something and cracked their tooth, and now they need a dentist. Or maybe they just moved and need to find a new family dentist they can trust. Regardless of the reason for the dental search, what comes next for the prospect is the desire to learn more.

Stage 2: Information Search

This stage is when prospects become more receptive to information and even tend to actively educate themselves.

Prospects are also generally more receptive to your paid ads and other marketing methods at this stage, such as your Google search results. Your goal is to get people to your website, which – as we've mentioned – is much like your home base of operations.

The big mistake here is trying to get someone to go straight from Google search to picking up the phone to call. While this can happen occasionally, most prospects will want to learn more about you before they commit. This is why your website is so important. It must educate prospects on *why* you are the best choice if you hope to sway them.

Stage 3: Evaluation of Alternatives

This is when potential patients process the information they have gathered. They may take time to evaluate and "rate" their options before making a buying decision. By this time, there are several processes at work inside the consumer's mind, including all the beliefs and attitudes about all the other practices they have to select from.

However, these processes all "evolve" based on a set of attributes the consumer is choosing to evaluate dentists by, whether that's the website design, procedure fees, the perceived value of treatments or services offered.

Stage 4: Purchase Decision

This is the stage where the decision has been made after careful consideration. However, this selection is not set in stone. A single negative online review or word-of-mouth trashing can still sway the prospect into another's dental chair.

Stage 5: Post-purchase Behavior

This is the stage when your patients face their second decision, whether they will remain a patient of their selected dentist. They will compare the services they have received along with their unique experiences and will decide if they are truly satisfied – or not.

This stage of the buyer's journey is of the highest importance when it comes to retaining patients.

Regardless of whether your patient is satisfied or dissatisfied, they are likely to share their feedback with others, either through online reviews or on social media. Some may recommend your services to a friend or co-worker. Therefore, it is vital to develop positive post-purchase communication with every patient in order to maximize your success.

Decision Attributes and Conversion Elements

You may be wondering how patients judge dental professionals. You are in luck. What follows are the elements most prospects and patients use to determine whether one dental practice is worthy of their time and attention over any other.

Hours

If your dental office is only open during banker's hours and your prospect is usually working during that time, you will lose that lead opportunity. On the other hand, if your office stays open late, on weekends, and during most holidays, scheduling an appointment with your office would be mighty attractive to a person with a full work schedule.

Services

Many patients would prefer visiting an office that offers a variety of services under one roof rather than be referred to a specialist in town. On the other hand, a patient may be more likely to visit your office for root canals if your office specializes in endodontics.

Ratings and Reviews

The office with more positive online reviews will draw the eye and attention of prospective patients more often than not. On the other hand, if your practice has a single raving review stating that you are the gentlest dentist in town, that might lend more weight to attract more patients than a practice with a dozen generic reviews.

Mobile-Friendly

A person viewing your website with a mobile device will have a tough time if your site isn't responsive. A responsive website is one that tailors itself to any sized screen. No matter if the person is holding an iPhone, iPad, or they're at work on their desktop, they should have a similar and *memorable* web experience.

Being responsive doesn't only mean that your content is easier to read, watch and view; that's a big part of it. But responsive sites are also laid out properly for the screen. The person doesn't have to do a lot of scrolling, because the "meat" of the page shows up front and center. Your phone number is easy to locate and submitting a question via web form or signing up for your newsletter is a breeze, even if the person is forced to navigate with over-sized fingers and thumbs.

Prospects will not tolerate a dentistry website that cares little for their web viewing experience.

They would rather visit a dentist that makes it easy to learn more about the practice and services, payments and insurances, your chair-side manner and how to contact you. Make it easy for your prospects, and they'll be more likely to schedule a visit.

Website Conversion Elements

Your website's goal is to secure leads for your business. You can think of your website as your "digital storefront." It should be visually appealing, easy to navigate, and must include multiple ways to get in touch. For best results, provide a unique offer, like a new patient special for under forty-bucks!

Phone Service

If prospects call only to be put on hold or if your office staff is rude and can't answer simple to complex questions, you probably won't close many appointments. On the other hand, if your team is friendly, knowledgeable and able to build rapport with callers, your schedule is more likely to be jam-packed from open till close.

Patient Service

When prospects become patients, they will judge your office with each interaction. This includes how they are treated at the front desk, how long they must wait, the level of the doctor's chairside manner, and how comfortable they are during various procedures.

But it doesn't stop there.

They will also judge how they are treated when it comes time to settle the bill, as well as on all post-appointment communications. In other words, doctor and staff should never let their guard down when dealing with patients, as quality patient service always matters.

Payment Options

Patients want to be able to settle their accounts quickly and easily. If they must jump through hoops, they'll feel let down. And if they find out that you don't accept their insurance after a procedure has been completed, they can become quite disgruntled. Experiences like these can contribute to poor marks and even worse word-of-mouth.

MULTI-TOUCH ATTRIBUTION

The following will provide you with a framework to help you better understand the journey new patients take to go from prospect to patient. You will also come to understand how each piece of your marketing strategy fits together.

Everyone's new patient journey is different, and multi-touch attribution is vital to understanding which pieces of your marketing efforts are working and which ones aren't. This is important if you hope to attract lifelong patients at your practice. Multi-touch attribution is about lending weight or value to each part of a new patient's journey.

As an illustration of multi-touch attribution, if you ask your patients how they heard of you, you probably won't get a single, clear answer. Most patients focus on the first or last touchpoint that led them to call your dental office. It is very unlikely that they will list their entire journey.

For instance, a patient may say that he heard about your dental office on Facebook. He won't go into detail, on the other hand, about how he originally heard about your services from a friend who then shared the Facebook page. That led the prospect to your website, to an ad on Facebook, and then back to your site where he finally picked up the phone.

So, don't be afraid to dig a little bit when asking, "How did you hear about us?" As you now know, a new patient's journey can be quite complicated.

The Whole Is Greater Than the Sum of Its Parts

Giving 100% of the credit of that new patient to his friend's referral is misleading. While that was the first touch attribution that eventually guided him to your site, you will eventually want to get as much detail as you can about the comprehensive journey that brought the patient into your office.

The first and last touchpoints – the ones patients often give you – seem like the best way to track your practice's marketing efforts because they are easy to understand. And sadly, this is precisely how most dental offices operate.

However, the new patient journey is full of multiple platforms, and several twists and turns. It typically covers more than one device and a multitude of marketing efforts. Therefore, the entire journey must be measured as a complete whole.

Multi-touch attribution can help you identify which combination of marketing channels or campaigns should be credited with each new patient.

On the following pages, we map out two different new patient journeys, so that you can visualize the multi-touch attribution framework.

As you can see, the new patient buying cycle looks overly simplified. And that is the idea. We have made every effort to make it easy to see how patients go from prospects to sitting in your dental chair.

The bare-bones of it is that they search online to learn more, visit your website and become better educated, then they call your office to schedule. But as we've established, rarely is the journey this simple.

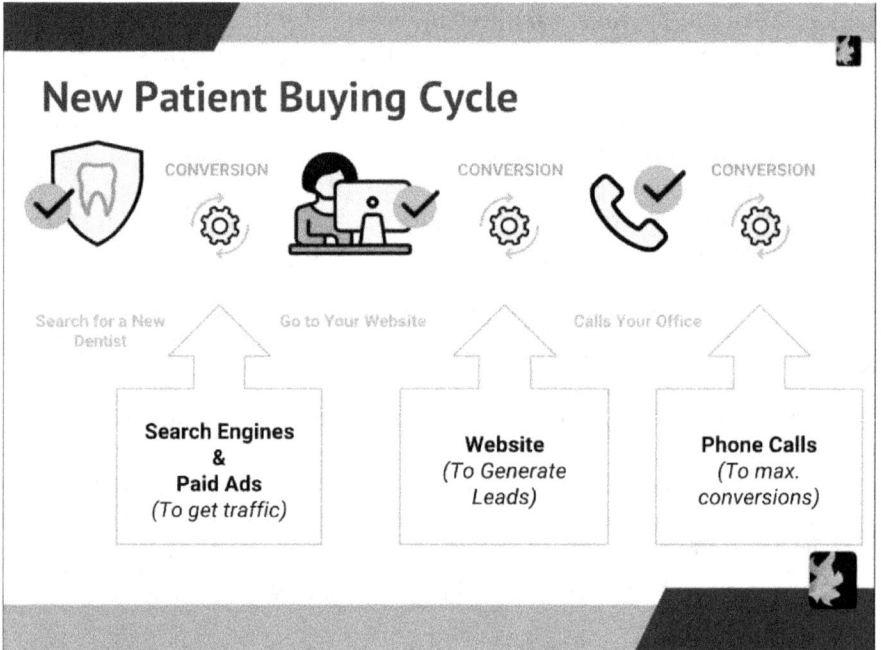

New Patient Journey #1

In this example, the patient hears a referral from a friend or family member, then searches Google for more information. After seeing your phone number in Google, the prospects calls to schedule an appointment.

That same prospect may not call after the initial search. Or maybe they called the office just to ask a question, but they didn't commit right away. That prospect may search Google for online reviews, but they still might not commit. It is only after the prospect has seen a few paid ads that they become enticed to click-through to visit your website.

After reading more on the site, such as a description of services and staff bios with plenty of smiling faces, that is when an online booking software can seal the deal, leading to the patient's first-ever appointment.

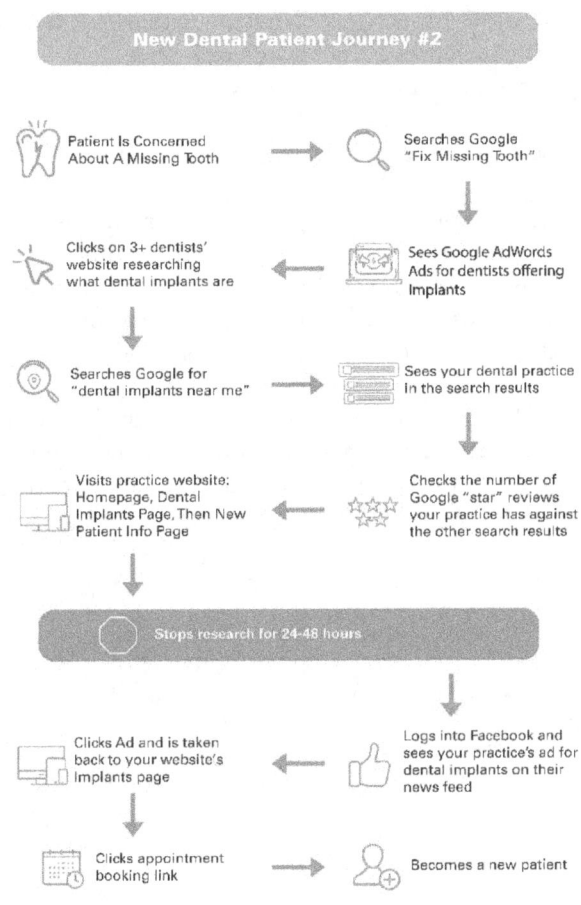

New Dental Patient Journey #2

In this patient journey, the prospect loses a tooth and feels distressed enough to search Google for "Fix Missing Tooth." Right away, the individual sees several paid Google AdWords ads for dentists offering dental implants. This takes the prospect on a journey through three dentists' websites. Even after all that, the patient doesn't decide.

It takes another Google search for "Dental Implants Near Me" to display your dental practice's website. The prospect then checks out your online reviews, visits your website to learn more, and…he still can't decide.

After that, the prospect gets distracted with life. A full two-days later, the prospect sees your ad on Facebook, visits your dental implants web page, clicks on an appointment booking software, and becomes an official patient.

Focus on Conversion and You Will See Results

In review, remember that prospects jump from many different aspects of your digital marketing campaign before they commit. This is why having a website or only relying on word-of-mouth is never enough. Every aspect of your campaign must be maintained and tweaked over time to ensure an efficient and memorable patient experience.

After all, these are real people visiting your site, seeing your ads, and calling your office on the phone. Your campaign must appeal to those individuals at every turn. That's where the marketing funnel comes in.

New Dental Patient Journey #2

- Patient Is Concerned About A Missing Tooth
- → Searches Google "Fix Missing Tooth"
- ↓ Sees Google AdWords Ads for dentists offering Implants
- ← Clicks on 3+ dentists' website researching what dental implants are
- ↓ Searches Google for "dental implants near me"
- → Sees your dental practice in the search results
- ↓ Checks the number of Google "star" reviews your practice has against the other search results
- ← Visits practice website: Homepage, Dental Implants Page, Then New Patient Info Page

Stops research for 24-48 hours

- ↓ Logs into Facebook and sees your practice's ad for dental implants on their news feed
- ← Clicks Ad and is taken back to your website's Implants page
- ↓ Clicks appointment booking link
- → Becomes a new patient

Multi-Touch Attribution pg. **6**

51

CHAPTER 5: THE MARKETING FUNNEL

While the buyer's journey is critical to understand, we feel it is also essential to explain the conversion funnel, otherwise referred to as the marketing funnel. This is the system we use to track the progress of leads from prospect to patient. Using the funnel system, we can more accurately identify what's working, what's not, and why.

The marketing funnel has three essential parts - the top, middle, and bottom.

Top of Funnel

The top of the dental marketing funnel is often called the "Awareness" stage. This is where prospective patients are considering a dentist, but they don't really know where to start. They may Google "Dentist in Phoenix," for example, to see what comes up.

These are individuals who may be in need of a teeth cleaning or root canal. They have an immediate need for a dentist but lack the awareness or trust to seek out a specific dental professional by name.

Prospects at the top of the funnel typically have the highest cost-per-acquisition, as you have to move them all the way from the top of the funnel to the bottom before they become actual patients.

The key at this stage of the buyer's journey is to position your dental practice everywhere a potential patient may look, including at the top of Google's search results. But patients may also look on Facebook, Yelp, or they may call a friend who recommends you, which then sends the patient to your website.

Getting found and noticed at the awareness stage of the conversion funnel is critical to building long-term brand equity with patients and getting more patient referrals. This is also the most difficult stage that requires the highest investment of time and money.

Middle of Funnel

This is the stage of the buyer's journey often known as the "Nurture" stage. By this time, the prospect may have been exposed to your brand one or more times. However, the person is still not convinced that you are the best choice.

To sway middle funnel prospects your way, you will need to use tactics like paid search marketing that keep your practice top-of-mind, encouraging the person to return to your site and call.

Tactics that work at this stage of the buyer's journey include retargeted ads, which track prospects across the web after visiting your website. For example, after visiting your site, your ads may appear on Facebook right in the prospect's newsfeed.

Email marketing re-engagement is also a tactic that is effective at swaying "on the fence" prospects. These are prospects who may have downloaded an ebook in exchange for their information but who then went non-responsive, for example.

Making sure your website is at the pinnacle of Google's search results for key local phrases will also help during this stage as prospects attempt to self-educate.

Most importantly, your dental practice should be listed on all local directories – and consistently – so that prospects can always find the most accurate business name, address, and phone number in order to learn more and schedule an appointment.

Bottom of Funnel

The above stages require more of a "Push" action on your part. You are pushing prospects into the top of the funnel and progressing them through.

At the bottom of the funnel is when prospects are more intentional with their searches. They know exactly what they want, and they have an idea who will be the best choice. This is often called the "Consideration" phase of the buyer's journey when prospects weigh their choice between you or the other guys.

Prospects at this stage of the buying cycle have the lowest cost per acquisition since they are ready to make a decision and have already gone through the awareness and nurturing stages of the conversion funnel.

Tactics that work at this stage include an internal referral program, AdWords and Facebook paid ads, and discount offers that attract new patients when your services are needed most.

Conversion Optimization

Everything we do is designed to remove roadblocks from the conversion funnel. That is, we try to determine why prospects aren't converting, and we repair the funnel until leads are being converted into actual patients.

From creating strong AdWords ads to getting our clients more Google reviews to creating an easy-to-use website that is appealing and helpful - and with clear calls-to-action - we make sure that your funnel is created properly and fortified at every turn.

However, we don't just look for things that are wrong. We develop our conversion funnels so that they are more effective for our clients, unlike other marketing companies.

For example, we help dental professional stress their differentiator options, such as same-day implants or a $39 new patient special. We use software that allows for website booking, completely eliminating the need for prospects to call. And we train your staff to be better on the phones, ensuring the highest patient close rate.

That last part is an aspect of the conversion funnel many of our clients don't consider at first. If they aren't getting new patients, the finger quickly gets pointed at the marketing company; the ones pulling strings behind the scenes.

Instead, the fault may be an employee who doesn't smile when answering the phones or who can't answer specific questions, such as how much you charge for dental implants.

Yet, whoever runs the front desk of your office wields an immense amount of responsibility. The person answering the phones and greeting patients is the literal face of your business as far as prospects are concerned. Therefore, the person must be polite, knowledgeable, and have a way with people that makes new prospects comfortable enough to schedule, and current patients satisfied enough to return.

You can track your website visits and newsletter conversions, but if your front desk staff can't close patients, your conversion funnel will then be known to possess a major flaw. Only when that flaw is corrected can we hope to get things back on track.

If you don't know what your staff's patient close rate is, that's equally as problematic, as then you won't be able to tell where your conversion funnel is broken at all.

The entire idea of a conversion funnel is to make it easy for prospective patients to find out more about you and choose you as their dental professional. After all, why make things difficult if they don't have to be?

That is why we advise dentists to look at their digital marketing campaign as a whole, including all calls that come into the front office. We call this 360-degree marketing. All the above steps - from the top of the funnel to the very bottom - must be analyzed thoroughly and repaired along the way for the system to work properly.

From hearing about you through the grapevine to clicking on Google, visiting your website, and calling to schedule their first appointment, your digital marketing campaign and staff must work in conjunction if you are going to maximize your success.

To put it simply, if your practice is struggling to find patients, digital marketing can help. But you must continuously analyze your campaign so that you can identify any weaknesses where your prospects may be turned off and pushed into the open arms of the competition.

To ensure that your digital marketing strategy has the most impact on new patient acquisition, here are a few questions to consider:

> **How do new patients tend to find you online? Is it through word of mouth or a Google search?**

> **What does a prospect find when landing on your website? Do they have their questions answered? Do they look**

around a while? Most importantly, are they enticed to return more than once?

- What is it like for a prospect to pick up the phone and call your office for the first time? What sort of welcome are they greeted with? Does the call leave them satisfied or wanting more?

- Are prospects ever put on hold? If they are, for how long? Is there music, silence, or are they treated to some kind of spoken message while they wait?

- Do prospects immediately schedule to come in for an appointment? If not, why?

- What kind of service do patients receive when they arrive for their first appointment? Dental exam, teeth cleaning, or emergency dentistry, for example?

Each of these interactions with your dental office has a profound impact on whether or not the patient will ultimately decide to visit your office and return for more.

CHAPTER 6: HOW TO OPTIMIZE YOUR PRACTICE FOR SUCCESS

Optimizing your dental office is critical to maximizing your digital campaign results. First, we feel it's important to discuss how communication has changed in the digital age.

The Realities of Modern Communication

If your staff is stuck in the past when it comes to communicating with prospects and patients, you won't go nearly as far. Instead, train your staff to keep the following *realities of modern communication* in mind at all times.

Immediacy

Technology has made people impatient. They want information now, not later. That means that putting people on hold and not being able to answer questions will quickly turn prospects and patients off. Instead, your staff needs to be quick with information and assistance if you hope to remain competitive.

Ubiquity

To attract new patients, your dental office needs to be everywhere new prospective patients tend to hang out online. The phone is still important, but it is not the only way to communicate with new leads. Your staff must make use of SMS text messages, chat boxes, web forms, social media, and automated appointment schedulers. In other words, your staff must be able to communicate using people's widely varying communication habits.

Knowledgeability

Not only should your front office staff be trained to answer the phones with finesse, but they should also know how to nurture new patient leads via email or in-office visits while at the same time retaining a five-star offline reputation through word of mouth.

The following steps will help to give your practice that boost and polish, so you can retain clients, maintain appointments, and create loyal patients for life.

How to Achieve Front-Office Efficiency

As you now know, the best online and offline lead generation strategies still won't bring you success if your front office isn't optimized for conversions.

FIREGANG FACT: Nine times out of 10, if your website traffic isn't converting prospects into patients, the issue is with your phones.

When it comes to conversions, the biggest missed opportunities are at the front of the office, where prospects and patients are greeted on the phone or in person.

You may be thinking that your front office staff already knows how to answer the phones and successfully convert new patient calls into appointments. We sincerely hope that's true. But we also know that, on average, the following *is* true.

- **30% of dental office calls go unanswered.**
- **Of those calls that do get picked up, only 50% get scheduled for new appointments.**
- **That means that if 20 people call, six of those calls will go unanswered, and only 7 of the 14 remaining will schedule an appointment.**
- **That's 13 missed opportunities!**

Think of all the potential revenue and growth you are missing out on if 65% of new calls are slipping through your staff's fingers! It's not exactly the front office staff's fault, but it does mean that additional training may be required to ensure growth and production.

To avoid this catastrophe, your dental practice must implement call tracking and recording. A tracking phone number will be placed on your website, for instance, so that we can track how many website visitors call your office. We can then record and listen in on the conversations your staff is having with prospects to fine tune as necessary. This mix of measurement data provides an easier way to identify which staff members are making the most of prospect opportunities as well as identify ways where additional training may be needed.

Ensuring that your office staff is optimized for conversions puts more money in your pockets with no extra expenditure! It's the difference between leaving things to chance and deciding to be smart about your digital marketing efforts.

If 11 leads call, but your office can only convert two of those prospects into patients, you'll only get an 18% return on marketing investment. Imagine being able to double or triple that number with a few staff meetings and training sessions. Numbers like that could have a dramatic impact on your bottom line.

How to Respond to Emails and Online Form Queries

Instruct staff members to respond to all practice emails in a timely manner. Your website should also include a form that allows prospects and patients to schedule an appointment or contact a staff member for additional information.

When an email arrives from a prospect, your staff should send an email right back. Don't sit on the email and go off to do something else. Immediacy shows that the prospect is a priority and that your office and staff care.

While it may be tempting to pick up the phone and call the prospect directly, some people may be at work and cannot talk on the phone. It is best to send an email and ask when the prospect is available for a phone call.

Email is somewhat intimate as a communication medium, but it doesn't hold a candle to the phone call or in-person visit. The ideal situation is to get prospects on the phone or in person as soon as possible so that you can connect using the human element. It is that very element that will convert prospects into loyal patients.

In-Office Visits—How to Meet and Greet Patients

Your staff should greet every person who walks through the door with an enthusiastic smile. For best results, use the person's name if you know it. If all representatives are currently assisting someone and another prospect or patient walks through the door, the staff should acknowledge the person with a friendly nod and let them know they will be helped in a moment.

For better results, offer the person a beverage and ask them to please make themselves comfortable in the waiting room. Just don't keep them waiting for too long.

When introduced to a new prospect, it is important to greet the person in a friendly manner and to address them by name. Ask how they heard about your practice, which will enable you to track where they came from. If the person was a referral from a current patient, make a note to thank and reward the referrer.

The overall goal is to make the new patient feel special and positively reinforce their decision to walk through the door. Make them feel as though they have come to the right place, that their search for a quality dentist is now over and that they are an important and welcome new edition to your dental office. If you can manage to convey those sentiments to every new patient who walks through the door, those individuals will be more likely to tell others about their positive experiences.

A typical in-office visit may go something like this:

New Prospect: Hi, I've never been to your office before, and I wanted to make an appointment.

Staff Member: That's terrific, I'm so glad you chose **[Office Name]**. What's your name?

New Prospect: My name is **[New Prospect Name]**.

Staff Member: It's great to meet you, **[New Prospect Name]**! My name is **[Staff Member Name],** and the doctor's name is **[Doctor Name]**. How did you hear about us?

New Prospect: My friend **[Referral Name]** told me.

Staff Member: Well, we're glad to hear that. We really love **[Referral Name],** and I'm going to make a note right now to thank her **[Or Him]** for bringing you in. I take it you want to schedule an appointment for a full oral exam and teeth cleaning. Why don't we begin by having you fill out a new patient information form? You can sit right over there and enjoy a hot cup of coffee while you fill it out. Here is the form. Please take your time and let me know if you have any questions.

Another in-office visit may go something like this:

New Prospect: I'm looking for a new dentist, and I've heard about this place. What do you charge for teeth cleaning?

Staff Member: Well hello! I am so glad you chose **[Office Name]**. What's your name?

New Prospect: My name is **[New Prospect Name]**.

Staff Member: It's great to meet you, **[New Prospect Name]**! My name is **[Staff Member Name]** and the doctor's name is **[Doctor Name]**. You said that you heard about us. How did you hear about us specifically?

New Prospect: I looked you up on Google, I think.

Staff Member: Well, we are very glad you did. We have put a lot of effort into our digital marketing presence to make sure that everyone sees how committed we are to professionalism and treating our patients with the very best in oral health care.

Now to your question. I'm glad you asked about teeth cleaning. We recommend that you schedule an appointment to meet **[Doctor Name]** so that he may provide you with a full oral health exam. Since your smile is unique, your teeth-cleaning fee may be different from another patient's. What dental insurance do you have?

New Prospect: I don't have insurance.

Staff Member: Great, less paperwork to fill out. Let's have you meet with **[Doctor Name]** as soon as possible. Why don't we begin by having you fill out this new patient information form? You can sit right over there and enjoy a hot cup of coffee while you fill it out. Here is the form. Please take your time and let me know if you have any questions.

Tips to Remember When Greeting New Office Visits

Always greet the person by name and acknowledge their presence, even if you are currently helping someone else.

Ask how the prospect heard about your office in order to track your marketing results. If possible, ask about their comprehensive buyer's journey. **(See Chapter 5: The Marketing Funnel)**

> ➤ **Get the person to fill out a new patient information form**

> ➤ **Ask about insurance and have the person bring proof**

> ➤ **Schedule the appointment immediately**

How to Nurture New Leads

Prospects who call, email, or step foot into your office are surely interested in your dental practice, but not every prospect who shows interest is ready to commit. This is where lead nurturing comes into play.

The trick to nurturing your leads is to contact them the moment they show interest and then to stay on top of them until they commit. We suggest that you rank leads according to their level of interest, with 1 being the lowest levels of interest to 3 being the highest, for example.

For example, a prospect with a ranking of 1 is not interested at this time. A ranking of 2 indicates that the person is somewhat interested, and a 3 means that the person is very intrigued by your office.

During regularly scheduled meetings with your staff, go over your leads, discuss any new prospect details, and alter their rankings accordingly. Then, schedule your leads for phone calls so that every morning a certain number of individuals are contacted for an attempted close.

The following script assumes that the prospect left a voicemail message and expressed great interest in the practice, explaining that he is looking for dental services for him, his wife, and three daughters.

Staff Member: Hello, may I speak to John Strauss, please?

John Strauss: This is John.

Staff Member: Hello, John! My name is **[Staff Member Name]** with **[Office Name]**. I wanted to thank you for leaving a message with our office. I understand that you are looking for dental services for your family. We are so glad you called. How did you hear about us?

John Strauss: I saw the video you posted on Facebook.

Staff Member: Oh yes, our Facebook video. We had a lot of fun filming that video. I'm glad you saw it. And it just so happens that I have the perfect appointment for you. Actually, I have two. You can bring your family to meet **[Doctor Name]** on Monday, December 8th, or Monday, December 15th. Which one works for you?

Three Tips for Nurturing Leads

1. **Train Staff:** Leads should be called as soon as possible. Aim for 24-hours or sooner for best results.

2. **Rank Your Leads:** Rank leads according to interest level and keep on top of leads that are closest to committing.

3. **Call Leads:** Train staff to set aside time to nurture leads daily.

Offline Reputation Management—Word of Mouth and Testimonials

The above steps that outline how to answer the phone and greet customers will help your practice improve. And when that happens, word will travel.

To encourage even more patients to spread the good news about your practice, here are the steps we advise our clients to follow to accompany the success of their digital marketing campaigns.

Steps for Improving Word of Mouth

- **Train Staff to be Friendly and Attentive:** With improved phone and interpersonal skills, prospects and patients will feel invited and welcome.

- **Put Some Personality into It:** Let your staff's personalities shine to make your office experience even more memorable.

- **Explain Everything to Patients in Great Detail:** Strive to help patients understand their diagnoses and the treatments that the doctor recommends. You should also explain billing and insurance procedures at this point. The patient should never feel as though they have been surprised or tricked when visiting the office.

- **Provide Amenities to Enhance Comfort and Well-Being:** A cozy waiting room with soft seating, magazines, TV, and tablet computers can go a long way toward making patients feel at home and ready to boast about your practice to anyone who will listen.

> **Available Treatments and Quality of Services Rendered:** The fewer times patients must be transferred to specialists and the more satisfied they are with your services, the better. Word of mouth will surely travel if patients can feel confident that the state of their oral health is always in good hands.

> **Patient Fees Match Perceived Value:** Work to ensure that the fees you charge match the value of the treatments your patients are paying for. In other words, patients should never feel as though they've been overcharged or ripped off if you want them to remain loyal.

Reviews for Marketing and Practice Improvement

We are going to show you how to use reviews throughout your digital marketing plan, but first you must earn them. We suggest that you get into the habit of asking patients for reviews following every appointment. Reviews also give you an opportunity to study and listen to your local market.

When you read the reviews that come in, keep in mind that - while good reviews are best - you shouldn't be offended if you get a few negative reviews. If you want to know precisely where your practice is weak and where you most require improvement, ask your patients what they really think about your practice and you will soon find out. You can then work on repairing any perceived flaws to improve your practice, reputation, and the results you receive from your marketing efforts, both online and off.

Reviews should be discussed with your staff on a regular basis, preferably during weekly or daily morning meetings. Let staff know the areas in which the practice needs to improve and seek to satisfy those patients who don't seem as happy as they should be.

How to Respond to Reviews

Here is a sample scenario that will describe how to respond to both positive and negative reviews for best results.

Review Example #1

"I loved my experience at Dr. Hanson's office. The staff was friendly and knowledgeable and my appointment seemed to fly by. I actually look forward to my next appointment." - **Katie J.**

Office Response

"Hi Katie, this is Joan in Dr. Hanson's office. Thank you so much for the positive review. We also look forward to your next appointment. We hope Johnny has fun during his first day of school!"

Notice how Joan not only wrote her name, but she referenced a bit from Katie's review and mentioned a conversation they had during the appointment. Make sure you don't reveal any private information so that you don't commit any HIPAA violations.

Review Example #2

"I just had a root canal by Dr. Hanson and I think my mouth is infected. I'm not happy." - **Anthony R.**

Office Response

"Hi Anthony, this is Joan in Dr. Hanson's office. I'm very sorry to hear that you are experiencing discomfort, but thank you for letting us know. Dr. Hanson is very thorough and will want to see you right away. Can you please call the office so that we can schedule an immediate appointment?"

This time, Joan still thanked the reviewer for leaving his thoughts, even though they were less than positive. Still, Joan offered to make the situation right, which can help to sway prospects who may be on the fence. It shows that your office cares, which is very important.

How to Respond to Facebook Comments & Reviews

Facebook is handled a bit differently than Google when it comes to reviews since it is a social network. In this scenario, notice how the patient is encouraged to share their experience further.

Facebook Review Example #1

"Dr. Smith treated my entire family to teeth cleaning yesterday and the appointment was so easy. From having playthings in the lobby that kept the kids occupied to the tablet computers that helped the appointment pass by, we had a very enjoyable experience. Would recommend." - **Janice H.**

Office Response

"Hi Janice, this is Mark in Dr. Smith's office. Thank you so much for the positive review. We really enjoyed treating your family yesterday. Dr. Smith said that next time, we'll be sure to have your favorite movie as one of the selections. Turns out, it's one of his, too! Remember, if you share your experience with ten people, you will receive ½ off Teeth Whitening."

In this case, Mark thanked the patient and mentioned something from the experience. He also gave the patient something to look forward to at the follow-up appointment. Finally, the patient was encouraged to share with family and friends for a treatment discount, which was first mentioned in the office and then reiterated on Facebook for all to see.

Facebook Review Example #2

"I wouldn't recommend Dr. Smith. He was rough, and my jaw still hurts from where he pulled my tooth." **- Sydney Z.**

Office Response

"Hi Sydney, this is Mark in Dr. Smith's office. Thank you for leaving the review. We are very sorry to hear that you are feeling discomfort. That can sometimes happen with a tooth extraction. We would like to schedule an immediate follow-up appointment. Can you please call the office so that we can discuss a time that would be best for you?"

In this response, Mark was very polite. He thanked the patient for her review and mentioned that the pain she is feeling can be normal. However, because the office cares, Mark is trying to get an appointment scheduled right away. The best-case scenario is that Sydney will be satisfied with that follow up, will change her review, and share the new, positive review with ten people to get a special discount.

How to Respond to Emails and Online Form Queries

Some patients don't like to talk on the phone and, likewise, are unlikely to make a public comment on Facebook. When a web form question or comment comes in, staff should respond first by emailing the prospect back. In this return message, staff should tell the prospect that the office will be in touch.

Here is a specific example of how to reply to a web form lead.

Web Form Lead Example #1

"Do you have wi-fi in the office?" **- Thomas Katz**

Office Response

"Hi, Thomas, thank you for emailing our office. Yes, we do in fact provide wi-fi. Not only that, but we even have tablet computers you can use to watch movies while Dr. Smith treats your smile. We can discuss all our amenities when you come in for your first appointment. Is October 1st or 13th best for you at 2pm?"

Web Lead Example #2

"Hi, I'm wondering if you can tell me how much you charge for a root canal?" - Susan Harrison

Office Response

"Hi Susan, thank you for emailing our office. Since every patient is different, we'd first want to get you in for a free consultation. That way, the doctor can determine the best treatment plan for you. Then we can give you a better idea of your final cost. However, Dr. Smith is very thorough and would like to examine your smile so that we can determine if a root canal is indeed the right treatment for you. Is September 13 or 23 good for you at 1pm?"

Key Takeaways When Responding to Reviews Online

- **Respond to the lead by name and thank the person**
- **Mention something from the review**
- **For negative reviews, ask to take the exchange offline**
- **For positive reviews, ask the person to spread the word**

Keeping Track of Reviews

Your office should be tracking all reviews that are sent follow-up responses. We have found that many practices use a spreadsheet where information can be easily separated, filtered, and recalled. The spreadsheet must then be updated each time a response comes in.

Of course, if your office made use of practice management software, this information could be added to the platform along with any notes that can be used to improve future communications. Software like this can also provide your staff with prospect names and numbers to call come morning, once the office has opened for the day. This method keeps leads on constant alert, ensuring that your office remains top-of-mind.

Get an office reputation your competitors will envy. Download your free reputation management guidebook at http://www.firegang.com/book-bonuses/

Converting Phone Calls into Patients

It is important for your front office staff - or whoever answers the phones - to understand that there is money involved just about every time the phone rings. The most obvious example of this is the new revenue generated by a new patient.

It is not so obvious where the money comes into play when a phone call originates from your website or an email, each of which relies on a different aspect of your marketing budget. Once understood, this process will help you focus on the areas where your marketing dollars are most effective while helping you generate the highest returns possible.

For instance, patient A may call your office after seeing your phone number on a dental referral website, while patient B may have searched Google for practices nearby, then visited your office to schedule in person.

Your practice gains revenue from every caller or visitor that is converted into a patient, so this is where we want to focus our efforts.

What follows are the fundamental steps we encourage you to enact to keep your bottom line in the black and your practice constantly growing and improving.

3 Keys to Front Office Success

Key 1: Always Go for the Appointment

The purpose of all phone calls is to book an appointment, period. Whether a caller asks about insurance, your office amenities, or driving directions, your staff should always be asking if the patient wants to schedule an appointment. Often, prospects are only a simple invitation away from visiting your office. The adage "you don't get what you don't ask for" holds true here. If your office staff doesn't ask for the appointment, you won't secure half as many won deals.

No Fee Discussions Over the Phone

Giving away fees during a call, even if the conversation is going well, can cause you to lose your advantage. The patient can now price check and undercut you, even if the other dental professional performs less-than-stellar work.

If your staff is giving away the goods too early, prospects can lose interest before they even know what's on offer, and why your service are priced the way they are.

It is far better to get the patient into your office for a face-to-face before you begin discussing fees, options, and treatment plans.

Use an Attractive Offer

You can get far more patients into your chair by offering an incentive to visit your office. A free checkup, discounted teeth cleaning, or similar discount or giveaway will encourage patients to book an appointment, especially if the offer is only available for a limited time.

Building Rapport with Callers

At this point, some clients want to know what happens when a caller demands to know what fees you charge or has an objection your staff can't overcome?

An untrained person might become rude or pushy in an effort to guide the caller directly into scheduling an appointment. This approach is counterproductive because it will only turn callers off, forcing them to call and possibly select one of your competitors for their dental health needs.

That is why your staff needs to build rapport, which is easier said than done. It's not impossible, you just need to know the right steps. Let's delve into those steps now.

The Basics of Dental Patient Rapport

Rapport is another way to describe a connection you make with a prospect or patient. In a traditional sales approach, rapport consists of spending a bit of time discovering the patient's needs.

This, again, is where clients want to know about the insistent caller. If the front staff is told to consistently go for the close, how are they supposed to focus on needs and satisfy the prospect all at the same time?

It can be done. It just takes finesse.

It is true that your front office staff should be taught to focus on "closing," or encouraging a caller to book an appointment at every turn. Doing so will maximize your conversions and ROI.

Unfortunately, this approach in the wrong hands can soon turn into a "get 'em in at all costs" philosophy, which can significantly degrade the patient experience. Constantly trying to close a patient without first building rapport will come across as cold and uncaring.

Instead, it is important to focus on the patient's needs while also guiding the appointment to a successful close. This is easier said than done.

You can begin by training staff how to answer all questions and address common concerns. They should know your insurance and payment policies, descriptions of your services, and be knowledgeable about dental ailments and symptoms.

Most of all, instruct your staff to always tell the truth. If a patient asks about a certain type of insurance and your receptionist dodges the question just to get the patient in, that will lead to a poor customer experience if you don't accept that patient's dental insurance provider.

You never want to give prospects or patients the wrong expectations, because that's when people tend to get angry and tell everyone they know - including anyone reading online reviews - that your office is to be avoided because you mislead and lie. Definitely not the outcome you want.

In contrast with the "get-'em-in" approach, the vast majority of your staff's time and energy should be spent establishing rapport with every caller. That is a prime way to set your dental office apart from the very first interaction.

Imagine a patient calls with a toothache. Instead of "Why don't you schedule an appointment right now?" your staff should ask what happened, and if the tooth hurts. Have they taken any steps to preserve the tooth and do they have dental insurance? These questions show that your staff member cares, and the patient will trust your office and be more open to booking an appointment.

FIREGANG FACT: Insurance, fees, and services aside, it's the dental office that makes them feel more comfortable that patients most want to visit. That starts with building rapport over the phone.

If your staff can be trained to establish a personal connection with each caller, closing the call will become an effortless endeavor, for the patient will basically self-close. Your dental office will simply become the most logical and emotionally-satisfying choice for that prospect because of the trust built by your front office employee.

Here are some tips to teach to your staff for building rapport with dental prospects and patients on the phone.

Ask the Caller's Name

Use the name of the caller in the conversation, as people love hearing the sound of their own name. Furthermore, using the person's first-name makes the call more personal, which helps to form an emotional connection. Only 1% of dental practices do this. Become a 1%er and remember your prospects and patients by name.

Paraphrase and Repeat

To show that you are paying attention, paraphrase and repeat back to the caller everything they just said, especially to remain empathic to their needs. For instance, "You just broke your tooth and now you're in excruciating pain? Yes, Sandy, don't worry. We can help."

Ask Positive, Open-Ended Questions

Never asked a closed question (Yes or No) when an open one will do.

For example, instead of asking, "Do you have dental insurance?" Ask "What kind of insurance do you have, Mike?" Instead of "Have you been to a dentist recently," ask "Tell me, Sara, when is the last time you visited the dentist?" Open-ended questions get the prospect talking, which further helps to foster an emotional bond.

Rapport is the key to success in business and life. The concept of making a connection with others in a professional setting seems simple, but actually doing it requires talent and skill. With enough study and practice, your dental office staff will soon learn how to build rapport with anyone who calls, emails or walks-in.

How to Answer the Phone Like a Professional

In addition to building rapport, you can get your staff more phone-conversion-ready by implementing the following techniques. You won't find any phone scripts here. We used to use scripts, but we found them to be too cold and robotic-sounding when implemented during a call.

Instead, we recommend using a "cheat sheet" that contains the verbiage your staff is most likely to use, a list of FAQs, and other information.

Keep these sheets near every phone in the office for ease-of-use and teach your staff to be more *proactive*. That is, they should be guiding the call to the ideal outcome, which is, of course, to ask each and every prospect if they wish to schedule an appointment.

The alternative approach is to be *reactive* over the phone, which is to answer a question or two and then hang up the moment there is resistance or an objection.

Your staff needs to learn frame if they hope to close the most calls. For even better results, make the process of improving your team's phone skills a contest or game, with actual prizes. Encourage your team to get better and focus on the positives of training. Only then will the skills and techniques be more likely to stick.

Answer with A Smile

People on the phone cannot see your body language, but if you have a smile on your face, the energy is conveyed through the quality of your voice. Something about smiling infuses the call with warmth and friendliness.

The alternative is to be monotone, which makes you sound more like a machine than a person. In other words, and as you can imagine, slouching with a frown on your face while on the phone is not what new prospects want to hear.

Instead, train your staff to smile throughout every phone call, as that helps to build rapport with callers. Practicing conversations in front of a mirror while smiling will help them sound more genuine.

Smiling and being warm is not the same as being passive. It is possible to smile and be assertive at the same time, and that is what is required if you hope to have a high patient close rate.

It's just a fact that prospects and patients need to be guided into setting an appointment. If Julie, who takes calls at the front desk, for example, isn't confident and doesn't speak with assertiveness, the prospect on the phone or the patient in front of her will naturally take control of the interaction.

On the other hand, if Julie is friendly, professional, and assertive, and at the appropriate time in the interaction directs the caller to make an appointment while proposing specific dates and times, the prospect will be more likely to schedule right there and then.

Ask If You Can Put the Caller on Hold (If You Must)

Callers tend to get upset if they are put on hold for more than 30-seconds. If you must put callers on hold, do it for only a moment, or offer to call them back as soon as possible. Consider using this verbiage, "**[Caller name]**, I want to spend time dedicated specifically to you, so I can answer all of your questions thoroughly. However, I am with another patient right now. When would be a good time for me to call you back so I can better assist you and give you my full attention? What is the best contact phone number for me to return your call?"

A Note About Phone Trees

Dentistry is a personal service, and patients expect there to be a live person on the other end of the phone. While phone trees can help with customer service in some industries, in our opinion they are bad for dentistry. We have heard dental patients directly state that phone trees result in a poor user experience. When you factor in robotic answering, long hold times, and the frustration of having to wait for menu items, most patients would rather hang up and call a competitor where they know a human will answer the phone.

FIREGANG FACT: Dental practices that remove their phone trees can increase their patient close rates by 15-20%.

Give your patients what they want, which is immediate service when they call. If you can't help them right away, call them back. A person would rather be called back than put on hold any day.

Ask if the caller has insurance

Make sure to ask about the patient's insurance information very early on during the phone call You want to avoid wasting time on the phone with someone who will decline to book an appointment because you don't take their dental insurance.

Train your team to be knowledgeable

In addition to knowing the office address and driving directions to your door, your team should also be trained on the basic descriptions of your services, current specials, the basics of insurance, and satisfying answers to frequently asked questions. For instance, if a prospect asks, "How long will my appointment take?" and "Do you take my insurance?" Your staff should know these answers without having to look them up.

The team should also be ready to address common objections, such as "It's too expensive," or "Your office is too far away for me." The less time you keep patients on hold or transfer them to find the answers to the questions they ask, the better. And the more the team practices overcoming objections, the more comfortable they will sound, and the more effective they will be when speaking with callers.

Never Eat or Chew Gum

Staff members risk turning callers off by chomping food or gum in their ears during a call. People tend to chew faster when they're nervous also, so your staff may not realize they're annoying callers until it's too late. Whenever the phone rings, staff should be trained to empty their mouths, smile, and answer while giving all callers their full attention.

Give the Caller Your Full Attention

When a prospect or patient calls on the phone, staff should be trained to pick up and refrain from doing anything else. They shouldn't type, read or send text messages. Instead, they should smile, answer questions, and guide the prospect toward the appointment.

If the staff member is not prepared to give the caller his or her undivided attention, it's better to let the call go to a carefully prepared voicemail message than to let the phone ring or put the caller on hold.

But what if someone walks in and the phone rings at the same time? This common situation can be confusing. Does your staff member serve the prospect on the phone or the patient in front of them?

Patients who walk in always take priority. Staff should never allow themselves to be distracted by trying to hold more than one conversation at a time. There is no quicker way to break a personal connection with a caller or patient than to be distracted - either on the phone or in person.

Take Information

The trick for your staff, and the sign of a phone expert, is to be able to build rapport while mining for information along the way. Too many dental staff members rush through their phone calls like they can't wait to get off the phone. They ask all this information up front in rapid-fire fashion, and that only makes callers feel like they're suddenly in a job interview.

You do need information from the patient, such as their name, phone number, dental insurance provider, dental history, and other details, but few people enjoy being grilled for info.

Instead, take time building rapport, then gather the necessary information. People tend to remember the beginning and end of an interaction, while the middle gets a bit muddled. That middle part is where the information gathering should take place.

After empathizing with the caller and satisfying questions and needs, then you can ask the pertinent questions. But again, don't come off as robotic or like you're trying to interrogate the caller. Be gentle, kind, and as though you're asking a new friend - "What is your name and how can I help, Susan?"

The questions most often asked during this stage of the call include:

- **What's your name? (Then use it often during the call)**

- **What's a good call back number for you?**

- **What appointment time is best for you, Option A or Option B? (Be specific! Instead of saying yes or no, they'll be more likely to select one-time slot or the other.)**

> **How did you hear about us?** If the person says, "The Internet," try to get them to be more specific. Google, Yelp, Facebook or your website?

Once you have the information you need, then tell the patient you can't wait to meet them and end the call on a high note.

Continued Training and Accountability

Many dental practices have tried phone scripting or training in the past, but the pressure to stick to the plan coupled with the lack of auditing often causes staff to deviate after a few months. Staff who were once great then become lax. We've seen it time and again. There will be a major spike in answered phone calls and closed appointments only for the numbers to drop three, six, or nine months later. This is explicitly due to the fact that there is no one holding staff accountable and rarely is there ongoing training. When staff revert to old habits, the whole practice loses.

That is why we recommend ongoing training with frequent refreshers to ensure everyone answering all phone calls properly. We also recommend constant testing and listening to calls to ensure staff never forget their training or stop trying to close as many appointments as possible.

How Long Does Training Take?

The longevity of any training program is subjective. Elements like employee turnover and timid employees can set training durations back months. That is why we recommend that doctors become accustomed to 24 to 36 months of partnership with their marketing company, at the very minimum.

Sadly, not every doctor feels this is beneficial. Many doctors want to partner for 12-months, but by month seven they are already looking for the next shiny object and falling for false promises by other marketing companies, regardless of how good their digital marketing campaign is performing. But without seeing long-term consistency, many doctors get jumpy.

If your company has excellent staff, each member can be trained by our team, and their phone calls honed over time thanks to tracking and phone monitoring. This is hands-on marketing that has made us a success many times over. Too many companies are set-and-forget, but that isn't how we operate.

We have real people checking reports, and phone calls are listened to and scrutinized by experts who know what to listen for. For instance, did the caller get a name, ask for insurance, and give the prospect at least one or two appointment times to select from? These monitored calls are the best defense against a conversion funnel that may have glaring holes.

If a new patient does not book an appointment, we can coach your team using specific examples so that we can show how to handle similar calls in the future.

Much of this advice doesn't come naturally but must be worked at and honed over time until it becomes second-nature. But once your staff becomes accustomed to always getting it right, you should see your conversion rates continue to rise.

Get a list of phone scripts to turn your front office into a goldmine. Visit http://www.firegang.com/book-bonuses/ to learn more.

CHAPTER 7: DENTAL MARKETING WEBSITE CHECKLIST

If you read the first edition of this book, you would notice that this section has been completely transformed. We used to advise dentists to take control of their websites by building it themselves. We no longer advise this, as home-made websites just won't cut it in today's digital age.

Instead, we advise that you have your website designed by professionals, either through your marketing company or by another web designer. Only by infusing your website with web and SEO best practices from the beginning can you hope to compete against, say, corporate dentists.

Web Design Best Practices

Visitors to your website will begin to judge the look and feel of your "home base" the moment it loads onto their screens. They will decide in just a few moments if your site looks clean and professional, or cheap and thrown together. The latter may cause prospects to click away and choose a competitor who does put effort into a stellar web-viewing experience.

How do you know when your website has been created by a web design professional who knows digital and dental marketing? What you need is a checklist. Check your site against the following points to determine if you are making the best first impression you can.

Simple Domain

Your domain name is your website's address. It is also referred to as your website's URL or Uniform Resource Locator. The domain name you select should be easy to say, type, and spell. We don't recommend using your name as your domain, such as "Dr-So-And-So.com." A personalized domain can make it difficult to sell your dental practice down the road. Domain names can become highly-valuable the more they age and starting over with a new domain can decrease the value of a business's website.

FIREGANG FACT: The closer you can get to a local search phrase with your domain name, the better. A great example of this is Anchorage Midtown Dental.

Easy to Navigate

Prospects and patients should be able to find the content they want within one or two clicks. Even if they have to use a search box on your site, that's better than having to search endlessly for information about root canals, for instance.

To make your website easier on prospects, have a prominent menu bar with drop-down menus of all sub-pages. For instance, a prospect may have to click on Services to find Root Canals, but at least the menu made it simple to find.

Secondary menus in your sidebar and tertiary menus in your footer can further guide prospects to the necessary areas of your website. As long as they don't add clutter to your website, added navigation can make your site even more user-friendly.

Responsive and Mobile-Friendly

According to Smart Insights, 80% of Internet users own a smartphone. Therefore, it's a safe bet that bet that most people visiting your website will be doing so on a small screen.

When websites were first created, they were built for desktops, which means that they could stretch from one side of the screen to the other. With all that space, webmasters were generous with their text, graphics, and layouts.

These days, you can't be generous with text, images, and layout on an iPhone screen, for example. All the elements will become jumbled, and you will make things very difficult with those with larger thumbs and fingers. Can you imagine trying to click a tiny link when the links are all jumbled together? A prospect would rather click-away and try a competitor than put up with a non-mobile-friendly website.

Earlier we mentioned that a responsive website is one that tailors itself to any screen size. You can test the responsiveness of your site by viewing it on a mobile device or by dragging your desktop browser window until it mimics a mobile screen. If the text and graphics meld themselves to the size of the screen you're using, your website is considered responsive, which is excellent for SEO.

On the other hand, if you must do an excessive amount of scrolling to find links and menus and such, your website is not responsive, and you will lose traffic. That much is guaranteed.

However, responsive is not the same as mobile-friendly or "Mobile First." Responsive merely means the screen becomes optimal for the device in the user's hands, but mobile-friendly means something different. It means to be cognizant of the fact that people will be using smartphones and tablets to view your content. They don't want to scroll or click too many times, and they expect to be taken directly to their intended locations.

For instance, if a visitor lands on your site and is immediately greeted with appealing graphics, short snippets of easy-to-read text, images that don't get in the way of clicking and navigation, and the highest-quality and properly sized media, they will be more likely to schedule an appointment. The thinking is that, since they had a positive experience on your website, they just may have a similar experience in your dental chair.

On the other hand, if your website requires excessive scrolling, your text is too difficult to read, and your images require people to scroll through someone's face to get to your web form, for example, that's too much to deal with for most mobile users.

Remember, people are impatient. A bounce rate is when people "bounce" from the home page immediately upon landing. Having a site that makes navigating on mobile a chore is a good way to get an elevated bounce rate, which tells Google your site may be poor.

Not only will Google reward your site if your bounce rate is low but putting mobile-users first is a great way to secure enviable rankings. As we've mentioned, Google made mobile-first one of its prime ranking indicators. Putting smartphone, tablet, and even wearable tech users as your primary targets is the way to go moving forward.

Easy to Read

Most content online is written for an eighth-grade education level. Incidentally, that is also the grade level the President's State of the Union speech is written in. What does this mean to you? It means that you should stay away from overly complicated words. Never use a complex word when a simple one will do. Endodontics can be mentioned, as long as you make it clear that you mean Root Canals.

This does not mean that you should "Dumb Down" your content. It merely means to keep things simple. Your web content should be written by a professional copywriter who knows the ins and outs of SEO. You can tell if your website was scribed by a professional if it contains short sentences and paragraphs, simple words and phrases, and subheadlines to break up content. Bulleted and numbered lists can also help to snag a prospect's attention.

Above all, the content on your site should be written in short, bite-sized chunks. Think of the content you see on Facebook or Instagram. No one has time to read a novel online, and few have the patience or the eyesight to stare at a block-of-text for any length of time.

Instead, your content should flow with a positive, purposeful, and professional message, not unlike the greeting a prospect would receive walking through your lobby doors.

Fast Loading

Your website should load within 3-5 seconds on all desktops, laptops, and tablets. You are encouraged to visit your site on a variety of devices to see how long the home page takes to load. Very few people will wait longer than five seconds. You can even test your website using a platform like https://tools.pingdom.com/.

Several Forms of Contact

A person should never have to search for ways to contact your office from your website. Your business name, address, and phone number (NAP) should be prominently displayed. In fact, using eye tracking software, we have found that people's eyes move in a Z-formation from the top left-hand corner of the screen over to the right-hand side, then down and to the left and then to the right.

This is the very formation you want to use on your website. Your NAP placed in the left-hand corner of your header will not be missed, but it also won't be missed on the right side. As the visitor's eyes move down and to the left, that is when you should introduce them to what you offer, such as a headline declaring that you are the local town's implant dentist. Then, when the visitor's eyes move to the right to complete the Z-formation, you should immediately hit them with a call-to-action, such as a web form with "Ask a Question or Schedule" written prominently overhead.

Of course, a layout like that won't work on a tiny smartphone screen. For mobile-users, your NAP should be prominent on the screen along with navigation to help the visitor delve deeper into your site. For best results, a button to contact you or schedule should be available without scrolling. The less work you make people do, the more likely they will be to answer your call-to-action.

In addition to a web form and phone number, consider adding live chat to your website, which gives web visitors a simple and fast way to get assistance when it is needed most.

Ways to Schedule

A call-to-action can ask prospects to leave a message or call, but there is one CTA that trumps all: Scheduling an appointment. We recommend that you make use of one of the many software programs out there that makes scheduling right from your website a breeze. This should be the case whether the individual is on a desktop or mobile, and for best results should be a one-click affair.

Banners with Sales Messages

Let web visitors know somewhere on your page if you have any special offers. These help to set you apart and will help to attract prospects who may be on the fence about choosing you as their dentist.

Photos & Videos

Prospects for your office rarely know anything about you or your dental office. Smiling pictures of doctor and staff can endear prospects to the office before they ever set foot in the lobby. Try to use actual photographs instead of stock photos. That way, prospects can build a personal bond with everyone in the office before their initial visit, making for a more memorable experience overall.

Before and after pictures can also work for treatments like braces, Invisalign, and full-mouth reconstructions. Just make sure you don't show any surgery, bloody, or graphic pictures. People don't need any reasons to be put off about going to the dentist. Instead, keep images bright, positive, and always looking their best.

If images can endear prospects to your office, a video is ten times better. Watching a video of the doctor welcoming prospects to the office is almost like meeting him or her in person. Likewise, with the staff. And a tour of the lobby is just like showing up for an initial appointment and getting a guided tour of the facility by a friendly staff member. As we will describe later, video reviews are also effective, as there are few testimonials better than those that come straight from the person's mouth.

Why Choose Us

Your website should be infused with differentiators. These are the elements that set your dental office apart from all other offices in the area. Do you have tablet computers as an amenity? Are you easy to find right on Highway 90? Does your dental office provide all services under a single roof? Are you a specialist in dental implants? Is your office open on the weekend for emergencies? Don't assume that your prospects know this information. It must be laid out clearly and explicitly in a manner that is easy to comprehend.

Reviews

Online reviews are paramount for getting prospects to choose you as their primary dental office. If you have gathered a lot of reviews on Google, ask your dental marketing company to showcase the best ones on your website. This is called social proof, and people will be more likely to fill out a web form or click-to-call if they know others have had a positive experience in your office.

Trust Emblems

Logos and emblems from association memberships, publications, and even news programs you may have featured in will help to lend your office an air of credibility, which also contributes to more follow-throughs on your calls-to-action.

Footer Elements

When scrolling to the bottom of your site, visitors expect to find everything they need to prevent them from scrolling back up. For instance, a menu of services, map to your location, appealing images, and trust emblems can help to drive conversions.

Frequently Asked Questions

Ideally, you will want to have all your prospects' questions answered before they email or pick up the phone. You can do this with your web copy, images, and videos.

Your web copy should greet your prospects with positive and engaging language. It should describe the office and amenities, services, and what sets you apart.

Information About Doctor & Staff

The About Us page is one of the most frequently visited pages on a dentistry website. The page should include bios of the staff and doctor, as well as engaging photos and videos. These are the individuals who will be dealing with, treating, and speaking to your prospects and patients. Why not have a virtual meet and greet before prospects even schedule?

The Importance of Having a Quality Website

While it is true that your website is your home base of operations that allows you to gather and capture leads, it is only one tool in your digital marketing toolbox. With multi-touch attribution, you may have prospects visiting your Facebook page, reading your reviews on Google, clicking your ads in Google and Facebook, and only then may they visit your site to schedule.

However, always keep in mind that no matter if a patient finds you in Google, or through word-of-mouth, and even if the person first saw you on Facebook and then watched one of your videos on YouTube, all roads will eventually lead to your website, making it your number-one lead generator.

CHAPTER 8: AN INTRODUCTION TO SEARCH ENGINE OPTIMIZATION (SEO)

We have taught you how to conduct the proper research to plan your digital marketing campaign, we have discussed multi-touch attribution and the marketing funnel, and we've covered how to optimize your office for success. Now it is time to cover the crux of digital marketing - Search Engine Optimization or SEO.

The History of the Search Engines

Search engines are nothing more than automated programs that organize the web and all its content for one single purpose: to help you find what you need. Yes, you.

Google cares so much that it has taken on the responsibility of sifting through the millions of websites, blogs, social media accounts, and other content that is being uploaded to the web daily. The end result is an easy-to-read Search Engine Results Page that delivers the most valuable and relevant search results as they relate to your query.

In order to deliver the most accurate results, Google and the other search engines use powerful algorithms, which are mathematical equations that are always being tweaked to accommodate the never-ending stream of content that shows up online.

Search engines have existed in some form or another since the '90s. Back then, sites were ranked primarily by their page content. In other words, keywords were the prime order of the day. By using the right keywords that relate to relevant search queries on their web pages, webmasters could almost be assured higher Google rankings.

Then, Google arrived on the scene at the turn of the century and introduced the world to Page Rank, which sought to categorize websites depending on their content and levels of authority within their given niches or categories. The higher the Page Rank number, the more prominently that site's pages would rank in the search results.

Page Rank was also able to be passed from authority sites to lesser-known sites by way of linking, thus giving those unpopular sites a rankings boost.

Back then, it was common for webmasters to meet in online chat rooms and discuss how to "best" the search engines. That largely still goes on today, though we also have blogs to read, and books to buy – such as this one – that help us understand how Google determines its rankings.

Google will give some of its secret sauce away, but not all of it. The rest comes from marketing research, testing, and taking risks that either pan out or don't.

Google doesn't give away its secrets because it doesn't want anyone learning and manipulating its search rankings.

But back then, when Google was still new on the scene, it didn't take long for webmasters to catch on to how the Page Rank system worked, and some shady characters tried beating the system in an effort to undermine the SERPs for their own benefit.

These crafty webmasters stuffed their pages with as many keywords as they could muster and collected links from authoritative sites by the dozens, hundreds, and even thousands in a desperate attempt to dominate the search results.

While this gaming of the system helped some webmasters shoot to the top of the SERPs, many of them earning tons of money in the process, Google soon learned that people were cheating. Needless to say, Google planned a swift crackdown.

Not only were these webmasters manipulating a system designed to help search users better navigate the web, but the "cheating" websites were generally of poor quality, even for the time.

In fact, most of these sites were nothing more than blank pages stuffed with one or two keywords repeated over and again. This is hardly what Google had in mind when it sought to categorize and deliver excellent content to the you, its valued user.

The fact that most of these cheating websites were of lower quality was not surprising. Most webmasters looking to cheat the system were searching for the shortcut to riches, and delivering eye-catching web design, informative and entertaining web copy, and all the other elements that go into delivering a memorable web experience wasn't something these scammers were willing to do.

The moment Google altered its algorithm, all those sites enjoying inflated rankings plummeted in the search results. Money was lost, businesses were ruined, and more than a few angry webmasters vented their frustrations about Google in the most popular Internet forums of the day.

SEO historians often describe this race to game Google's system as a dance. Each time Google releases an algorithm update designed to thwart unscrupulous websites, those webmasters study the changes and inevitably develop innovative ways to beat it. This "dance" has gone on since the beginning of Google's search engine reign.

Google Gets Proactive

Then, around 2003, Google stopped resisting and started helping. For the first time, the search giant offered tips and suggestions for attaining the top positions for relevant keyword terms. And Google has continued to do so ever since via Google Search Console, its section of tutorials and advice provided to help webmasters. We will discuss and use Google Search Console in an upcoming section.

During that time, Google taught webmasters how to research the best keywords to satisfy user searches; how to attain backlinks, those links that lead from other sites to your site; and how to achieve relevancy through online relationships.

Over the years, Google has adapted to accommodate every new technology and user trend so that they can deliver the highest-quality results. For instance, in 2010, Google announced that it was using social signals in its search results, which is an indication that your target audience is sharing your web content on social media.

The search giant continues to fight against what is now referred to as black hat SEO tactics, those methods that are used to undermine and manipulate the system, and Google has consistently altered its algorithm ever since. New algorithms are released without warning and no one knows exactly how each one works. Google sometimes releases snippets of information to webmasters, but most algorithm changes are considered top secret. This undercover tweaking process usually halts the cheating, at least until some black-hatter comes up with new tactics to boost rankings without having to do any work.

People still try all sorts of ways to cheat Google, such as keyword stuffing, buying thousands of backlinks, purchasing social media connections, and by scraping content, a process in which content is copied and then slapped onto a lower-quality site to attain higher rankings. Google is watching, which is why you should never use these unsavory methods.

Follow the techniques outlined in this book and explore Google Search Console to absorb Google's instructions for using its search engine for maximum benefit. By aiming for gradual and consistent results with the proper use of keywords, building your links slowly and organically over time, and providing your visitors with the best experience possible, you can be sure Google will reward you.

Google Updates and the Resulting Aftermaths

Every year Google updates its algorithms, mostly to correct minor flaws. Examples of this include the Panda and Penguin updates, which decimated the rankings of sites that were relying heavily on backlinking.

Backlinking used to be a staple of SEO. The idea was that if an authority website linked back to your website, your site must be of the highest quality. The problem is that too many webmasters tried to manipulate the system, leading to inflated rankings. Google responded by making backlinks less relevant for SEO. Websites affected by this update took years to recover.

Rank Brain and AI

The latest algorithm changes involve futuristic technology that is truly "out of this world." Artificial intelligence (AI), for example, allows machines to learn much like humans do, and the implications are limitless.

Google is now using the Rank Brain algorithm, which uses AI to improve the user experience (UX). The new algorithm uses machine learning to make the search results more refined, trendy, accurate, and appealing.

In other words, with this new technology, Google almost knows what you want to search for before you do.

Mobile First

A while ago, Google announced that it would reward websites that were considered mobile-friendly. With smartphone, tablet, and other mobile searches becoming more popular, Google has shifted its focus to capturing more "on the ground" data while using it to provide more personalized and intuitive search results.

This is another reason why it pays to employ a digital marketing company, a team that has a vested interest in keeping up with Google's latest changes. While Google tends to keep its changes hush-hush to prevent people from cheating the system, analysts rush to study their algorithms, and we follow these studies carefully, as should all companies worthy of your time and attention.

After every Google update, there is constant online chatter from people claiming that Google destroyed their businesses or even their lives. You can usually trust that these people have succumbed to the temptation of black hat tactics and the promise of immediate and substantial gains. When it comes to SEO, easy come, easy go. Businesses that try to cheat Google tend to tank quickly in the rankings following a new algorithm update.

Ranking Without Breaking the Rules

Sites that use white hat SEO tactics, on the other hand, typically see no change or very slight changes when a new algorithm update is released. This is because the sites in question were doing exactly what they were supposed to be doing: helping site visitors become more educated, informed, and entertained.

Through the years, Google's updates have taken on many monikers, like Panda, Penguin, and Hummingbird. Each one comes with a different set of parameters that webmasters must take into consideration.

At the heart of all these Google algorithms are automated bots that regularly scan or "crawl" the millions of webpages, websites, and other content online. These bots, also referred to as spiders, will analyze your website looking for certain *signals*.

What do Google spiders look for? They analyze the colors of your site, the load speed, and the content and keywords you have provided. Most of all, spiders want to know if people have shared your website and its content on social media. Popular content, after all, must be quality, and so tends to rank higher than not-so-popular content.

Your website information is then indexed accordingly and presented to users as search rankings. Google uses more than 200 signals to determine the quality and relevancy of the various web pages online. If you can display soothing colors, engaging content, blazing-fast site speed, and all the other elements Google spiders are looking for, you just might achieve SERP dominance.

We have already provided you with many white hat SEO tactics for ranking prominently in Google, but in this chapter, we will go a bit further. Instead of going through the extensive Google Search Console library, we are going to do our best to break down the process of SEO in an easily digestible manner for you.

The steps you are about to learn come straight from Google and are considered legitimate, ethical, and the proper way to stay in Google's good graces. To begin, we are going to break down the typical search results page.

The Anatomy of Search Engine Results Pages

To view the SERPs in action, search for a keyword, such as "dentist in Altus Oklahoma," and see what Google retrieves and displays.

When the results come up, you will notice that there are two types of listings: paid listings and natural, or organic, listings. The organic listings are the ones we have focused on up to this point.

You can get a boost in the organic listings by including the proper number of keywords written naturally (no keyword stuffing!), and by ensuring relevant and quality backlinks are pointing to your site from authoritative websites.

Some excellent advice for webmasters who wish to remain white hat is to focus on providing your site visitors with the most valuable and memorable web experience possible. Do that and Google should reward you.

If you don't want to go through the trouble of optimizing your website organically, there is always paid online advertising.

Since Google search is a free service, many wonder how the search giant makes its money. Allow us to introduce you to Google's AdWords platform, which happens to be one of Google's primary revenue sources.

About 5,860,000 results (0.62 seconds)

Dentists Near You | We Work With All Insurance | aspendental.com
[Ad] www.aspendental.com/Dentist ▼
Schedule Your Next Dentist Appointment Online In 3 Simple Steps Or Call Now.
Online Appt Scheduling · 20% Off General Dentistry · Peace of Mind Promise
⚲ 8660 SW Scholls Ferry Rd, Beaverton, OR · Open today · 9:00 AM – 7:00 PM ▼

Local Tigard Dentist | See our New Patient Specials
[Ad] www.tigardfamilydentist.com/ ▼ (503) 506-2170
Family Oriented Dental Services. Schedule Your Appointment Today!
Accepting New Patients · Care for Whole Family
⚲ 11960 SW Pacific Hwy, Tigard, 97223

Best Dentist In Lake Oswego | Come See For Yourself.
[Ad] go.lodentalstudio.com/ ▼
We'll provide you & your family the best care possible. Schedule a visit today!
High Tech Dentistry · Financing Available · Top Lake Oswego Dentist

You can cut in line to a first-page ranking as well as reap all the benefits that come from such an honor if you're willing to pay for it. We will cover paid online advertising in greater detail in an upcoming chapter, but for right now, just understand that advertisers can bid for the top spots displayed for relevant keyword terms. With optimized ads and a healthy ad budget used intelligently, you can put your dental services in front of decision-makers who have a high likelihood of converting.

Ideally, you will want to reach the top spot of Google both organically and through paid advertising. Just consider what would happen if you suddenly had an influx of traffic coming from paid and organic listings. You could potentially double, triple, and even quadruple your business and income. That is certainly possible with enough time, attention, and search expertise.

How Google Ranks Dentists

Mobile Optimization

As previously mentioned, Google rewards sites that make the mobile-viewing experience a positive one. This is where having a responsive website is crucial. A person shouldn't have to scroll just because they're on a mobile phone. Your website should be tailored to all devices.

HTTPS Encryption

In 2014, Google announced that it was going to reward websites that secured its content with HTTPS encryption, which makes use of an SSL 2048-bit key certificate to keep your site safe from hackers. Sites that employ HTTPS tend to experience a significant boost in the SERPs.

Keywords

Google will search through your site to determine which words or phrases are repeated most often and rank your site accordingly. Therefore, you must use specific keywords when writing your online content, especially any pages that have to do with your business, location, and specialization. The key, however, is to write naturally. Do the research and provide unique content, but also use keywords and related keywords throughout, such as Endodontics, root canal, dental crown, dental treatment, and other terms users might be searching for in Google.

Longer keywords tend to be more specific and are easier to rank for, such as "Affordable dental implants in Birmingham, Alabama" but be careful about using keywords exactly as you suspect searchers might use them. Never sacrifice quality to appease Google.

Here's another way to put it. For best results, your content should be written for your ideal patient, first and foremost, but you should always keep Google spiders and what they most they want in the back of your mind.

Relevancy

Google must determine which sites offer the most relevant solution to any given user's search queries. Using the proper keywords in strategic locations can help immensely in this regard. So can writing content that speaks to the reader's emotions. Content that teaches a lesson or offers a unique take on a common problem also tends to do well. For best results, visitors to your site should feel it accommodates them and serves their needs better than anyone else in your space. Tough order, but with enough research and work, content like that can be created and served up fresh for Google spiders to crawl.

Legitimacy

Google has the tough job of determining if your site is an actual, valuable contribution to your audience or if it's merely a scam-site looking to rob people blind. You can help Google decide by providing excellent graphics, content, and useful information.

Authority

While crawling your website, Google attempts to determine its value. A valuable website should not only look, feel, and read the part, but it should be visited often and shared far and wide. Sites like those stand out, and Google tends to reward them.

Public Perception

Many clients feel that this is one area that is out of their control, but you can contribute to the way the public views your office using digital means.

You can begin by creating profiles on third-party platforms like HealthGrades, RateMDs, Kareo, and Wellness.com. This is a change from the advice we used to give clients only a few short years ago, which was to put their profiles on sites like Yahoo and InsiderPages.

While those sites are important, dental-specific sites will help to target your audience, which is exactly what you want. And if you can get more positive reviews on those types of sites, public perception will improve - and that is directly within your control.

Now that you know how Google ranks dentists, it's time to go back to the beginning. We're talking a trip back to where Google started all those years ago, by examining the keywords your practice uses to entice prospects to become patients.

Keywords—the Foundation of Internet Marketing

We have mentioned keywords a few times already, but this is an area of SEO that is rife with confusion. SEO has always been about keywords. These are the words Google users enter in the search box to find the information they need.

"Dentist in Austin" for example is a keyword an Austin dentist may want to use when optimizing his site. That means to place that keyword and variations of that keyword throughout the site's content, which tells Google to rank the site for queries related to Austin dentists.

Strictly speaking, the term "keyword" refers to a single word. When search engines first launched, they had relatively simple algorithms, and most users entered single words for their queries. But as search engines have evolved, they have grown to support long-tail key phrases with two or more keywords.

Long-tail keywords are also more helpful for users since they can now express their needs more precisely and Google can provide them with more relevant results.

Consider someone driving and using hands-free speech capabilities. A search for a dentist may be said as "Find me a dentist in Austin." or "Find a dentist near me."

Keyword Phrases

High-quality content using phrase-based keywords will work best on Google's search engine. The term "quality content" can be subjective, but it's one of those things you can always pinpoint.

Generally speaking, quality content is relevant, useful, and memorable, which is no small feat to create. We recommend that you hire the services of a web copywriter who is well-versed in SEO to create your content for you.

To find the ideal keywords so that your site ranks prominently in Google, you must know how your prospects are searching for you. Most people won't search for "endodontics" for example. They'll instead search for a "root canal."

Still, having both endodontics and root canal peppered throughout your content - along with other variations, such as "root canal treatment" or "root canal procedure," for example - will help your site rank higher for those types of queries.

Your keywords may change over time, which is why it remains important to keep your finger on the pulse of your target market.

If your competitors are using "root canal" and "tooth implants," and you're only using "dental implants" and "endodontics," you might not get noticed by new patients.

How do you know which keywords to use? Research, and lots of it. Using Google Trends, for example, can tell you what Google users have been searching for by area, time frame, and on various platforms, like YouTube.

Keep in mind that you should never rest on your laurels when it comes to keywords. It helps to consistently research the top keywords for your services and industry every six months. Search trends change drastically, sometimes due to pop culture influences, other times due to breaking news or changes in technology. Only by conducting the proper research can you hope to remain competitive year after year.

As you will soon see, there is an art form to proper keyword research and placement. Let's examine that art form now.

Three Keyword Types for Dentists

Since the beginning, we have focused our marketing efforts solely on dental practices. And in our experience, there are three primary types of keyword phrases for dentists.

Services

These are the terms that describe the various services your practice offers to patients, and how they help with various ailments, issues, and needs. Keywords in this category include Invisalign, root canals, cavities, and dental implants.

Insurance Coverage

People considering your practice may want to know if you accept their dental insurance. Insurance-related keywords include Aetna, Blue Cross/Blue Shield, Medicaid, and Humana.

Geographical Area

Google will provide you with more targeted traffic if you use keywords that mention the state, city and suburb names (and zip codes) that represent your service area. As a dental professional, you rely heavily on local customers, so including geo-based keywords is the perfect way to attract more of your neighbors to your dental office.

Which types of keywords should you use in your content? We recommend that you use all three types for best results.

Now it's time to research your ideal keywords like a Google SEO expert.

Keyword Research Tools

Google Trends (www.google.com/trends)

This free tool from Google will allow you to enter your keywords to trends of rankings from past and present. You can also view related keyword searches and regional activity, as well as a few other important details. This tool is great for narrowing down your keyword list.

5-Minute Site Tool (http://5minutesite.com/local_keywords.php**)**

This free tool allows you to compile a list of local zip codes and neighborhood names and is ideal for gathering the proper geographical keywords for your dental practice.

SpyFu (www.spyfu.com**)**

This tool costs money, but there is typically a free trial. Designed for pay-per-click (PPC) paid advertising campaigns, SpyFu can tell you what keywords your competitors are ranking for and which ones are the most viable for search and PPC dominance.

SEO Tool Set (www.seotoolset.com/tools/free_tools.html**)**

With both free and paid options, the SEO Tool Set allows you to enter up to 12 keywords at a time to see how they rank and how viable they are for your online marketing campaigns.

Google AdWords Keyword Planner

Considered the pinnacle of keyword tools, Google's proprietary keyword research client is reserved for AdWords customers only.

The Basics of On-Site SEO or How to Optimize Your Website

To get your website found in the Google SERPs, you first need to optimize your site for local relevance. The term "dentist" alone won't be tailored for local. "Austin dentist," on the other hand, will be.

You can also optimize your web presence for local searches by including images of your building's exterior, and then geotag those images using a site like http://www.geosetter.de/en/. This makes your site - and all of the images on your site - easier to find in Google's search, Google Image Search, and Google Maps.

Here are a few other ways to improve your on-site SEO.

Relevant Local Pages

Creating pages for your website that mention local landmarks, the history of the area, and even state, city, and county news stories will work.

Longer Keyword Phrases

The term "dentist" is a highly competitive keyword. Can you imagine how many Google results you would get back after searching using a term as simple as that one? A ton, as you'd essentially be telling Google that you're looking for a dentist in every location throughout the country.

Longer keyword phrases like "Dentist in Austin that accepts BlueCross," for example, are much less competitive and will yield more significant local results. Longer key terms also help users find what they're looking for easier, thanks to intuitive AI.

When Google spiders crawl your site looking for valuable and relevant information, they typically do so from the top down. That is how we will approach this next section. Starting from the very top of your website (known as the header) all the way down to the bottom of your site (known as the footer) we are going to teach you how to optimize your website internally. This process is known as on-site or on-page SEO.

Metadata

Back before content management systems like WordPress existed, websites had to be coded mostly by hand. To provide valuable information to your audience and appease the search engines simultaneously, you needed extensive coding knowledge to ensure you had the proper metadata, design, text, and videos that people could experience, read, and see.

Metadata consists of internal code that is explicitly designed to be read and processed by search engine bots, spiders, or crawlers (these bots have different names depending on the search engine you are referencing). Thanks to WordPress and plugins like Yoast, entering your metadata is as simple as typing it onto the page.

Title and Description Tags

The first pieces of important metadata that search engines will read consist of the title and description tags. Incidentally, these are the titles and descriptions that you read when you conduct a search engine query.

To see these, conduct a Google search and examine the first organic link that shows up on the SERP. The title is the part you see in blue, and the description is directly underneath it.

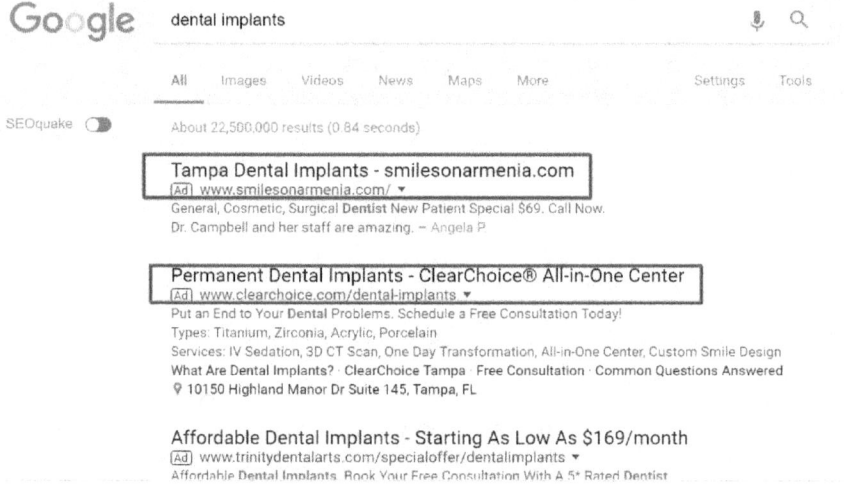

By manipulating the metadata within your website, you can determine what Google displays to prospects and patients when they conduct a relevant search.

You will want to write title and description tags for every page on your website. WordPress and Yoast make entering meta-data a no-brainer, as the data boxes appear directly underneath the space to create new Posts and Pages. However, you should never enter metadata quickly or without serious consideration.

Writing meta titles and descriptions requires time, knowledge of the field, and precision if you hope to increase your rankings long-term.

To begin, select Pages in the left-hand pane of your WordPress dashboard. Then, choose Add New. Or, if you want to write the metadata for one of your existing pages, select Pages and then find a page you have already created. Next, choose Edit underneath the page's title.

This action will bring you to the WordPress Page Creation or Edit screen. If you scroll down past the main content box, you will notice a Yoast section.

This is where you will enter your title and description tags, as well as the keywords you want to be ranked for.

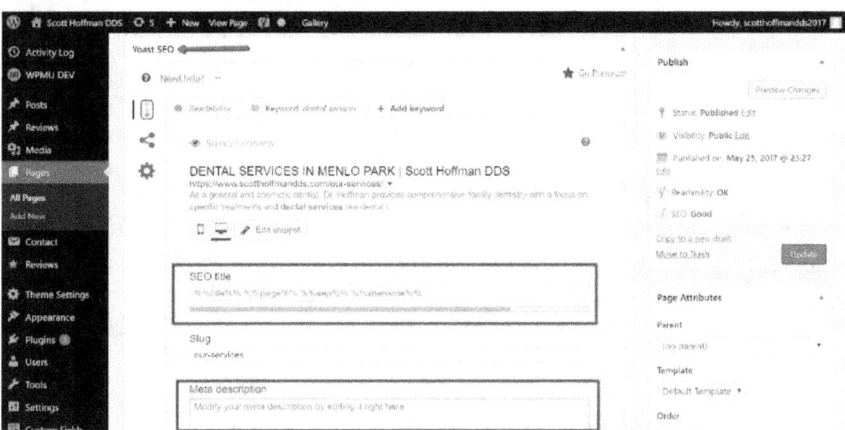

The metadata you enter will then give Google and the other search engines the necessary clues on how to rank this particular page.

How to Optimize Title and Description Tags

We recommend that you keep ever page URL and associated data on a spreadsheet for easier organization and retrieval. This same spreadsheet file can help you write and organize your title and description tags.

Your page title tags should include the name of your practice and at least one of your primary keywords. For best results, we recommend inserting geographic keywords in every title on every page. Shoot for fewer than 70 characters for best results. To check your character count, do a Google search for a free letter/character counter and enter your title tags to check their length and validity.

Dental Practice Example | Premium Dentistry in Austin | Most Insurance Accepted

Your description tags should include information about your practice and entice search users to act. For best results, include your phone number or other contact information. These should be 300 characters or fewer.

For example: Visit **[Dental Practice Example]** today and experience premium dentistry in a calm and soothing environment. Call now: 444-0111!

While it is important to use your keywords in your title tags, it's not as critical to use them in your descriptions, but every bit helps. Just make sure that your titles and descriptions are accurate, legible, and that every single one is unique. The search engines hate duplicate content, and you will be penalized for copying content, even from your own website.

Media Tags

The next meta tags that are crucial to your website's optimization consist of image and video tags (and all other media tags). Keep in mind that the search engines aren't just interested in the text on your website's pages. They are also concerned with the images, photos, videos, and sound bites. And luckily, WordPress makes setting and forming your media tags very simple.

First, click on Pages and Add New in the left-hand pane of your WordPress dashboard, or click Edit under the title of a page that you have already created. Once you are in the creation or editing page, you will notice a small button at the top left corner of the screen that reads Add Media. Click it.

Here you can upload media from a drive of your choice, or you can enter the URL of a media file from elsewhere on the web. Once you select your media, you will be directed to enter specific data about that media file.

Here is where you will set the media file's name or title, a caption, alt text, and a description. Name the title of your media file after your keywords. If you just uploaded an image that depicted a dental implant on the dental implants page, your title might be dental-implants-austin-tx.jpg.

We recommend that you name your media files just like that, with small letters and space separations for simpler identification and organization. We also recommend organizing your media files and their metadata attributes on a spreadsheet file just like you did with your page titles and descriptions. In other words, record and keep track of everything for easy recall later.

The caption you enter will show up on your web page underneath the visible file in question, and we advise you to use keywords in your captions for further on-page SEO. Your description of the above example image might be, "Dental implants: a viable alternative to dentures for our valued Austin patients."

Alt text is the text that will show up on text-only browsers or that will be read aloud to the hearing impaired. Remember, the search engines can't see your images and videos. They can only judge their relevancy by the metadata that you enter.

Your alt text should describe your images and videos and should include your keywords for best results. See the image below as an example.

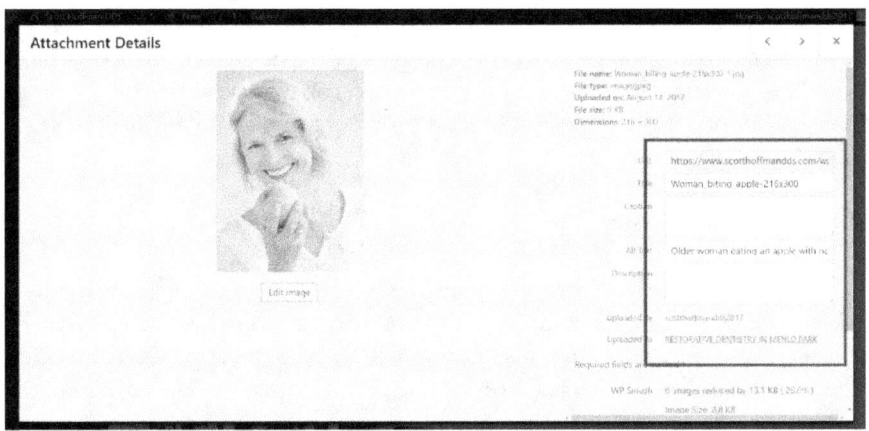

The description you enter will be used in search engine image searches. You should write this in the same vein as your page descriptions. Your example might read, "At **[Dental Practice Example]** in Austin, Texas, we use the highest-quality and most realistic-looking dental implants. Book an appointment today!"

Optimize all your media files this way, and you will surely get a leg up in the SERPs for all relevant searches.

Header-Tags

When you write the text content for pages, remember that our recommendation to break up the content with bolded subheaders and bullet points wherever possible. This makes the page easier on the eyes and the material much smoother to digest, while also improving SEO.

When you separate your content with bolded subheaders, use relevant header-tags. You can select these by using the paragraph drop-down box in the page editor.

Using Heading 1, Heading 2, Heading 3, and so on for your headings and subheadings will tell the search engines that those terms are crucial and thus should be considered when ranking your site in the SERPs. Therefore, for best results, use your keywords in your header or H-Tags whenever possible.

For instance, right above a paragraph about dental implants, we might use the Heading 1 attribute to write the heading, "High-Quality Dental Implants—The Best in Austin," assuming that those terms represent one or more of your primary keywords.

The H1 heading has a much higher importance in Google, so every page should have an H1 tag that uses the keyword for that page. It should be as close to the top of the page as possible. For best results, never use the same H1 twice.

Low Keyword Density

We mentioned that inserting your keywords into your web content is crucial for achieving high rankings, but we also cautioned against keywords stuffing. Your job is to use just enough keywords to appease the search engines while alleviating them of doubt that you are trying to game the system.

For best results, we recommend using your keyword in your page's title, once in the first paragraph, once in the final paragraph, and a couple of times throughout the page (utilizing H-tag keywords whenever possible).

This should provide your page with a keyword density of 1-3%, which is ideal for on-page SEO. To find your keyword density, calculate the word count of the page you have written and then count the number of times your keywords were used. Divide the keyword number by the word count to find your keyword density. Your calculation may look like this: 5 keywords/500 words = .01 or 1% keyword density.

Keep in mind that you may be using multiple keywords on a single page. To get the best results, you should calculate keyword density for each keyword that you use.

Internal Linking Structure

An internal linking structure is crucial to make your website more user-friendly. Visitors to your site don't always want to click on your main menu to find the content they want. When they stumble across particular keywords in your web content, such as dental implants, they may appreciate a link to your implants page. Not only will providing internal links make your site easier to navigate, but it will also help the search engines determine which keywords are the most important for ranking.

An internal linking structure also keeps visitors on your website longer, which is very good for SEO.

To create internal links, edit one of your existing web pages or posts and find a keyword within the content. Highlight the keyword and click on the Link icon in your page edit toolbar.

You will be taken to a pop-up page that asks for the preferred link URL. Here you can either enter a new URL if you want to provide an external link or you can search within your pages to provide an internal link. Since you are creating an internal link, you will want to find the page on your site that is relevant to the keyword you have just selected, such as your dental implants page.

The rule of internal linking is to keep it to one or maybe two internal links per page, depending on the word count. More than that may make your page too cluttered.

You should also make sure the pages you link to are relevant to the keyword in question. Ask yourself if linking to that page will make your site more user-friendly or if it will only lead to frustration for your web visitors. Remember that your goal is to help visitors navigate your page more efficiently, so approach internal linking with that in mind.

Site Map

Even though Google spiders can crawl your site and all of its pages in a matter of seconds (or perhaps fractions of a second), your assistance in helping them find what they need will usually be rewarded. One way to help is to give them an easy-to-crawl sitemap.

A sitemap is a coded document that showcases every link on your site in order of its importance. The idea is to give spiders or bots an easy way to go from link to link and page to page, ensuring they are able to analyze everything there is to index and rank.

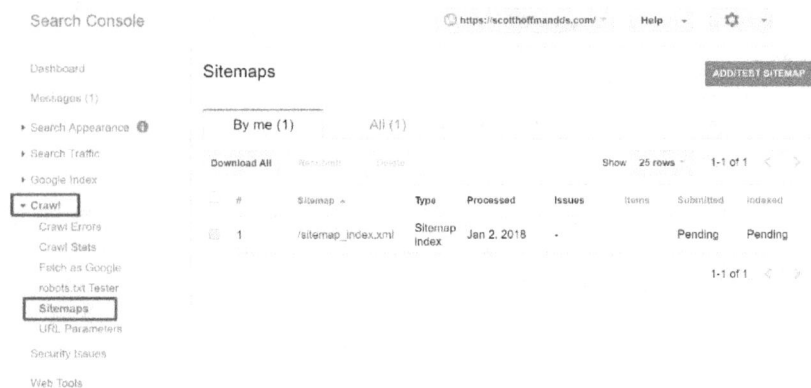

Creating a sitemap for your website is easy with the help of a site called XML-sitemaps (www.xml-sitemaps.com).

All you have to do is enter your website's domain name, the frequency with which you want the search engines to crawl your site, the last modification attribute, and your priority preference. Click Start, and you're off to completing your on-site SEO.

We recommend that you only enter your domain, hit start, and keep all the other options in their default positions. Once you have this document, you should submit your sitemap to Google Search Console. This tells Google that your site is ready to be indexed.

Keep in mind that, due to the steps we have already taken, Google will crawl your website even if you don't submit it to the search engine for indexing purposes. By submitting your site to Google Search Console, you are taking a proactive step that tells Google that your site is ready for indexing now rather than later.

Visit Google Search Console (https://www.google.com/webmasters/tools/home?hl=en)

Enter your website when prompted. Once your site is set up, click on your website name, then under the heading Crawl, locate the Sitemaps link.

In the upper right-hand corner, you will see a button that says Add/Test Sitemap. Click on that button, add your xml sitemap, and you're done. Well, almost.

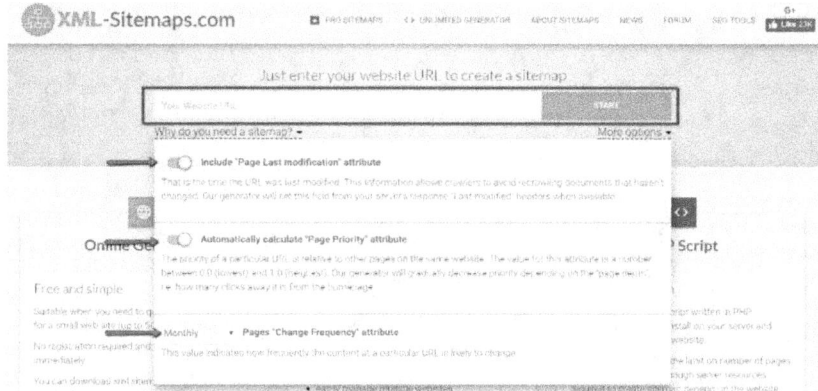

We also recommend that you place your sitemap in the footer of your website, which will make it easy to find for visitors and search engines alike.

Most footer plugins make it easy to insert your sitemap and other elements into your footer, such as social buttons and links that are important for legal reasons, like your Privacy Policy and Terms and Conditions.

A Final Word About Quality

We've already emphasized that quality content is relevant, useful, memorable, unique, and authoritative.

As an example, look at one of our clients, Anchorage Midtown Dental Center, which is a dental practice that hosts a patient education section on its website. There, patients can get answers to their frequently asked questions and learn more about what makes the office unique. Competitors who aren't doing this are missing out on this chance to make yet another personal connection.

The information on AMDC's website is informative and easy to digest. It also includes videos for prospects who don't feel like reading. The videos are short, filled with relevant information, and designed to do one thing - present the doctor as the absolute dental authority in the area.

Off-Site SEO—Establishing Authority

The first step of off-site or off-page SEO is to create a profile for your business on Google My Business, which started out as the social network Google+.

Google started Google+ to compete with Facebook. When those ambitions didn't take off as expected, Google+ was converted to Google My Business. As you can imagine, Google is invested in its social network and wants you to be, too. Therefore, being listed on Google My Business can help you rank higher on Google Search and Google Maps.

While Google My Business can offer prospects important information about your business, such as your hours of operation, phone number, and office address, and help you rank higher for local dental searches, Google Maps will give prospects turn-by-turn directions right to your door.

Make sure you have no duplicate listings on Google My Business. If you have two listings, your rankings could become confusing, which can then damage your ranking statistics. Google loves fresh, unique content, and will heavily penalize sites that copy content or provide poor-quality material.

When completing your Google My Business listing, you are encouraged to populate your profile with as much information as Google allows. Don't leave any spaces blank.

FIREGANG FACT: If you don't create a Google My Business listing, Google may still list your business, but the information may be inconsistent or incorrect.

NPI Registry Site

Remember how we encouraged you to create a website so that you can control the information disseminated across the web? Off-Site SEO is no different. While you can't control Google or any other third-party site, you can control what information is presented on those sites by creating profiles on prominent platforms.

The NPI Registry (National Provider Identifier) allows you to decide what information is distributed across the web as it relates to your business.

If you don't fill out a profile on the NPI Registry site, you have no idea what information may be distributed to dental and health directories across the web. Those platforms may be showing outdated phone numbers, inconsistent addresses, and incorrect services that can steer prospects wrong, and ultimately harm your reputation.

While you are filling out your profile, either on Google My Business or NPI, be sure to include plenty of smiling photos of doctor and staff. A few photographs of patients, their families, and shots of your office can add a personal and inviting touch.

Take care when completing your directory profiles, as these platforms can help you present your office as the go-to dental office in town, no matter where prospects may look online.

Off-Site SEO Vs. On-Site: Which is More Important?

Some will tell you that off-site SEO isn't as important as on-site. However, you could have perfect on-site SEO and still not be getting the rankings you hope to achieve. That is because Google and the other search engines are wary of sites that have excellent on-site but poor off-site SEO.

Off-site SEO, to the search engines, means that others vouch for your website. It represents social proof, and without it, Google and the other search engines may ignore your site altogether, no matter how perfect your on-site SEO happens to be.

Search engines use two primary factors when determining social proof: backlinks and social sharing.

Backlinks, as you now know, are external links that point from other websites to yours. For example, the local Chamber of Commerce linking to your site means that your site must have a decent reputation in your local community. Social sharing indicates that others have shared your website with their social followers and friends.

The more relevant your external links and the more your site is shared on social media, the more your rankings will climb, as long as those links and social shares were obtained legitimately.

Again, Google and the other engines are wary of sites that gain too many backlinks in rapid fashion. Similarly, you can get penalized or banned for suddenly accumulating thousands of social followers and shares seemingly overnight. To avoid sending up a red flag and to remain in Google's good graces, gather your links and social activity organically, which means bit-by-bit and over an extended period of time.

Three Tips to Improve Off-Site SEO

Contact Partners and Relevant Organizations

If you belong to the American Dental Association, the Better Business

Bureau, the local Chamber of Commerce, or other respected organization, contact those entities and ask them to link to your website from their sites and social profiles.

Social Sharing

Place social buttons on your website to make it easy for visitors to share your content on Facebook, for example. Many WordPress plugins can do this for you. You can also improve off-site SEO by sharing your pages and posts on your own social accounts, where you can encourage others to pass your content around.

Review Sites

Platforms like Yelp, Angie's List, and FourSquare invite others to review and rate businesses just like yours. It is important to be listed on these sites and to have some activity. While we encourage you to focus on Google reviews first, these other sites should be worked on after you have a solid Google rating to round out your online reputation.

Watch for Upcoming Google Changes

Google changes its algorithm 400 to 600 times every year. Each tweak is designed to deliver the most accurate and quality results to users while pushing the scammers and poor-quality websites toward the latter pages of the search results, where few ever venture.

That means that no matter how well you do or how much focus you put into your campaigns, you will always need to be keep adjusting if you hope to keep up. Missing one or two Google tweaks is acceptable but missing 400 to 600 every year can cause your website to plummet in the rankings.

Wait, You Have to Do This All on Your Own?!?

Right now, you may be thinking that all of this digital marketing stuff seems overwhelming. We don't blame you. Search engine optimization, social media, paid marketing, and all the rest that goes into an online campaign is a full-time job. It's not something you can do on your off times or weekends, especially when you are attempting to run a busy dental office.

Hiring a marketing company to oversee your website, SEO, and entire campaign as a whole will keep you on track to reach your digital marketing goals. A company can also keep up with the latest Google changes and latest techniques so you don't have to.

While do-it-yourself SEO can work, we don't recommend it. There is far too much to keep up with and learn, and too many changes to monitor in this ever-evolving field. Stick to what you do best, which is serving your patients, managing your staff, and growing your practice, and leave the search engine optimization to the experts.

CHAPTER 9: LOCAL SEARCH ENGINE OPTIMIZATION

The previous chapter was designed to give you the basics of what a search engine like Google may look for when ranking sites. We also talked about how to rank locally using keywords and geotags. These elements are critical for a dental office since you are primarily looking for local prospects. It's unlikely that people are visiting your office from across the country, for example. Instead, you have prospects searching "Dentist in [Your Area]. Those are the prospects we want to focus on now.

The search engines, and Google in particular, have been putting much focus into local search for quite a few years now. If you are searching from a desktop or laptop computer, Google will detect your location and do its best to yield local results whenever possible. And with GPS devices in most phones and mobile devices, providing search customers with local results is even easier.

As a local SEO professional, your job is to tell Google and the other search engines exactly where to rank your website so that your practice shows up for relevant and localized prospects and patients. This is where local SEO comes into play.

How Local SEO is Different

To see how a global search result looks, try searching Google for the keyword term, "dental staff training jobs."

Notice how Google delivers results from all over the web. You might even notice a video or two that could have been filmed and uploaded from anywhere.

Now look at what happens when you enter a geographical modifier into the mix. This time, conduct a search for "dentures in Austin, Texas" and note how Google not only yields results from Austin, Texas, but even provides you with a map so that you can gauge which dental provider is closest to where you live.

Entering your physical location, such as your city, state, and suburb is only half the battle when it comes to local SEO. The true determination of how well you rank locally depends on your use of *citations*.

Citations and Local SEO

A citation is a snippet of data that the search engines use to learn more about your practice, location, services, and hours of operation. At its core, your practice's citations consist of your Name, Address and Phone Number (NAP).

Take a look at your search results for the Austin, Texas, dentist. Notice how Google provides you with those doctors' names, addresses, and phone numbers. Those are citations at work.

It is crucial that your citations are correct and consistent across the web. Just as the search engines crawl your site for information, they are also crawling millions of other sites across the web from all over the world.

Ideally, you will want your practice's citations to be listed on your own website and other prominent websites, such as the Better Business Bureau, Dunn and Bradstreet, and your local Chamber of Commerce.

The more citations you have listed online—as long as they are correct and consistent—the more clout your online presence will have and the higher you will rank in the local search results.

Mapping Services

In a moment, we are going to teach you how to build your citations across the web. However, this information can be tedious and time-consuming. Due to the increased chance for human error (consistency of data entry is critical), we don't recommend building your citations on your own. We don't even recommend passing the task off to staff.

Having your citations prominently displayed in hundreds or thousands of places online not only makes your practice seem important, it makes your practice very easy to find for prospects and patients who may be using mapping and GPS services to find your office location.

Before you start to build your citations across the web, you need to make sure any platforms that currently list your practice are showcasing the most accurate information.

The platforms to check include Alignable, Citydirect.info, Thecityof.com, Localsaver.com, and Nextdoor, which are all local directories with high domain authority.

Getting listed on those websites with a backlink pointing to your website can help you rank more prominently and will put your listings in front of local prospects searching online for services just like yours.

Once again, we don't recommend conducting citation analysis and data entry all on your own. But even if you have hired a marketing company to do the work for you, knowing this information will allow you to check your company's performance and assess the progress of your campaigns over time.

Step 1: Check Your Citation Information Across the Web

If your practice has any information listed on one or more online directories—and chances are that it does if you have been at your location for some time—you are likely to find inconsistencies.

For example, Yelp may display an incorrect phone number and address if you recently moved locations.

To find out whether the information listed on the web is correct or not, we are going to recommend an important platform called MOZ. There is also a Google Chrome browser extension called NAP Hunter created by Local SEO Guide, which will yield similar results.

Moz (https://moz.com/local/search)

Moz allows you to search for your business name and zip code, then determines if your site is verified by prominent platforms like Google and Facebook. If your business can't be found, Moz will educate you on where to start listing your business. Sites like Acxiom, Citysearch, Facebook, Factual, Foursquare, Google, Localeze, Superpages, YP and Yelp will help your business spread its listings around. When it comes to listing your business – your name, address and phone number (NAP), you must be consistent. Any variation in your listings can cause confusion across the web, and your local rankings could suffer.

Step 2: Correcting Citations with the Big-Three Data Aggregators

If your listings can be found on any of the above directories, but there are duplicate listings and incorrect data, those errors will need to be fixed immediately. The longer they remain, the longer it will take for your local rankings to recover and start showing positive and steady results.

It is not enough to fix your listings on a single platform. Once you conduct a search using Moz or another Citation finder, you must go down the list and fix all of your listings one-by-one. That is the only way to ensure sites like Google and Facebook have the information you want them to have.

If you have just run a citation report and you have found your citations on a few online directories, social networks, and other sites, you may wonder how the information got there if you didn't submit any of it yourself.

Online directories like MapQuest, Yellow Pages, and even Google My Business "scrape" your practice information from authoritative sources, and those sources are where you should start if you want to control, correct, and maintain the most accurate information online.

If online directories had a hierarchy, the top of the hierarchy would be dominated by the three biggest data aggregators. If you have any information listed online and you didn't enter it yourself, chances are that it came from one of those three sites.

Let's examine the "Big Three" now so that you can edit any information that needs to be corrected before you proceed.

ExpressUpdate (http://expressupdate.com)

Visit ExpressUpdate to add or edit your site as instructed. Once completed, you will receive an email when the listing is considered "In review."

If you have a duplicate listing on ExpressUpdate, you will have to fax the organization with a duplicate removal request on your company's letterhead to (402) 836-3993.

Acxiom (www.acxiom.com)

You can check your business listings on Acxiom by visiting the Business Listings Manager page. You will be asked to search for your business by phone number in order to claim and correct any information listed. Do that and you will then be able to edit your practice information or add your business for the purposes of mass aggregation.

If your listing shows up but is incorrect, you won't be able to conduct a simple edit. Instead, you will need to add a new listing with the correct information. Register with Acxiom and follow the steps to submit a utility bill or proof of business registration.

After your listing is claimed and correct, you should delete all others so that there is only a single listing of your dental practice.

Localeze (www.neustarlocaleze.biz/directory/search)

When you land on the Localeze site, you will be asked to search for your practice by your business name and zip code or your city and state. You also have the option of searching by phone number.

Whether you add or edit your information, you will be asked to verify your listing by phone, just like you did with the other two aggregator sites.

If your information cannot be found on Localeze, you can add your information by buying a True Identity subscription for $79.00 per year.

Once you have finished adding or correcting your information on the "Big Three," your information will soon spread to many more online directories, social media sites, forums, and platforms across the web. Don't quit now: To be extra thorough, move on to the next tier of aggregators to further improve your local SEO authority.

Factual (https://www.factual.com/)

Factual refers to itself as The Leader in Location Data. The site brings together mobile marketing, digital consumer products, and real-world analytics to help brands get found by local searchers.

To update your information in Factual, you can add or edit your information using the online submission form. You can also go through

Trusted Data Contributors, which is a paid service.

Going through the submission form can take two or three months, and you will need to give Factual your 10-digit unique ID code so that the proper listing is being updated.

NPI Registry (https://npiregistry.cms.hhs.gov/)

The NPI Registry is a government-provided, free directory that collects all active National Provider Identifier (NPI) records. The platform is the main data source for all leading health and dental directories. The platform assists healthcare providers with a way to identify themselves in a standard manner throughout the industry.

Searching the NPI directory for your listing is a straightforward process. Simply add a few fields and hit Search. If your listing shows up and is the same as it is listed in Google, you will be good to go.

If your information is not listed in NPI, you will have to apply for a Type 1 NPI, which is for individual providers or Type 2, which is for organizational providers. You can apply using the form provided on the website.

Step 3: Inspect Other Key Online Directories

Your MOZ report will likely show the following sites. We recommend that you start with these before you proceed to any others if you want an accurate and consistent web presence.

Google My Business (https://www.google.com/business/)

By now, you should have already created a Google My Business profile, which – as we've stated - is critical for showing up on Google Maps and can contribute to higher rankings in Google local search.

If you didn't create a profile or you found a profile already, you may be witnessing information that Google has "scraped" from other sources. That is the very reason you need to claim your listings on authoritative sources if you hope to control, correct, and maintain the most accurate information online.

If your business does not populate on Google My Business, and you didn't create a profile when prompted before, you can create a listing here: https://www.Google.com/business/.

If your listing shows up on Google already, you will have to claim and verify that the information is correct. Otherwise, anyone can edit a listing on Google, and you don't want anyone to be able to control your information.

To claim your listing, you will have to follow the steps, whereby Google will send you a postcard in the mail containing a specialized code. Once entered, your information will be verified, which signals to Google that you are satisfied with the information and that, by all accounts, the listing is correct.

Your Google listing will show up in Google's search results. Therefore, you will want to optimize your listing every way possible. Begin by populating every field and including as many geotagged photos of your office as you are allowed. You can also add the URL to your appointment setting software so that patients don't have to visit your website at all.

Google Posts will allow you to bolster your Google My Business presence even further. You can post relevant content that excites and engages your audience and drives them to your website and office.

Google even allows you to create a Google My Business website, which is already optimized for mobile and ad-ready. The service is completely free and is one more way you can engage with prospects and patients. A Google-created website will give you an extra citation, and Google will quickly index it. This is recommended even if you already have a website in place. Google even allows for Live Chat functionality, which allows your staff to engage with patients directly anytime they need help.

Linkedin: https://www.linkedin.com/

LinkedIn is the world's most popular professional social network. Being found on LinkedIn is a great way to establish yourself as an expert in your field and can be helpful when it comes to meeting contacts and making connections within your industry. You should not only create a profile on LinkedIn, but a company page as well. All you need is a domain-related email to create a company page. If your listing already exists, you can claim it with the help of support. Follow the steps similar to how you verified your information on Google.

Apple Maps: https://mapsconnect.apple.com/

Apple collects its data from Factual and Yelp, but you can claim and update your listing by registering with Apple Maps connect. The platform's customer support is extremely helpful as long as you provide them with all the verification sources they require.

Glassdoor: https://www.glassdoor.com/

Glassdoor connects headhunters with jobseekers, but the platform also acts as a business directory. Adding your dental practice to Glassdoor is a simple affair. All you need is a domain-related email. Make sure you optimize your profile like you did on Google and others by filling out all available fields with relevant and quality information, and by adding geotagged images of your location.

Nextdoor: https://nextdoor.com/

This is another directory that is quickly gaining ground online. The process of getting a listing verified and updated on Nextdoor is fairly simple. Follow the steps and make sure your profile is optimized properly.

Bing Places for Business (https://www.bingplaces.com**)**

Bing is the second most popular search engine in the world. Owned by Microsoft, it hasn't quite gained ground thanks to Google. Google has become synonymous with search and has even become a verb for searching on the Internet. However, Bing is still used by quite a few people, and you wouldn't want to lose any prospects by ignoring the search engine altogether.

Similar to Google My Business, BingPlaces is the search engine's business directory. Complete your profile just as you did with Google My Business. Unlike Google, BingPlaces has excellent customer support, which will walk you through the creation, verification, and even removal of duplicate listings for a complete and accurate Bing profile.

Yelp (http://www.yelp.com**)**

Yelp helps people find highly-rated local businesses. The platform is also where people can go to leave a review about a particular business, such as your dental office. Creating a profile on Yelp invites others to leave their reviews about your services, and that is a very good thing, as most people today view online reviews as being as trustworthy as a personal recommendation.

Yellow Pages (http://www.yellowpages.com**)**

Remember those big yellow books people opened to find local businesses, addresses and phone numbers? Today, people in search of contact information simply have to visit yellowpages.com. Make sure your business is listed and correct so that customers can find you. Most of all, claim and update your listing so that any other aggregators receiving information from this ultra-respected online source have the correct information.

Super Pages (http://www.superpages.com**)**

Similar to Yellow Pages, Super Pages is another online directory that is still used by many humans and aggregators alike.

Angie's List (http://www.angieslist.com**)**

A cross between Craigslist and Yelp, Angie's List makes finding a specialist easy by offering profiles, advertisements, and online reviews for many local businesses. Many people use Angie's List to find dental professionals, so don't leave Angie's off your list of databases and review sites to use.

Angie's List has undergone a complete remodel as of late. To join Angie's List, which puts businesses like yours in front of interested prospects, visit https://office.angieslist.com/app/join.

Local Stack (http://www.localstack.com/san-diego-ca**)**

This site advertises that customers can find local businesses in half the time. Of course, your site must be listed for that to happen. Luckily for you, the process for claiming, adding and editing your information on Local Stack is easy. You will also be pleased to know that many local TV stations use Local Stack to provide data for their Yellow Pages sections.

Local.com (http://www.local.com**)**

If you look at the bottom of Local, which is a very prestigious local data aggregator, you will notice that it reads, "Some data provided by Acxiom," which you may recognize as one of the big-three data aggregators online. Your data may already be correct on Local since you added or edited your site on Acxiom, but check your information on the platform just to be sure.

Kudzu (http://www.kudzu.com**)**

Kudzu mentions that it gets most of its information from Localeze. Again, check to see if your practice is listed on Kudzu just in case.

Yellow Bot (http://www.yellowbot.com)

Yellowbot is important, especially because some local directories such as businessfinder.nj.com use their data.

Yellow Book (www.yellowbook.com)

When you add your information to Yellow Book, prospects and patients will be able to find your phone number, address, and a map to your location. They can also click a link that enables them to receive a call from your practice.

If you need to update or edit your information, simply send your update request to Yellow Book support, and the staff will update your data quickly.

Four Square (https://foursquare.com)

This platform allows users to check-in and leave reviews while visiting your office, all from their smartphones. Foursquare is a very important player in our mobile-centric world. People share their tips on various places, such as dental offices, and they can even check-in to tell others they've arrived for their appointments.

Foursquare can even be connected to Pinterest Maps. Not only that, but Google really seems to favor FourSquare. You can easily claim your profile on the platform by calling support to manually verify your listing. You will need to upload some sort of verification documentation, such as proof of signage, an exterior view or utility document. Once received, support will approve your update request.

Merchant Circle (http://www.merchantcircle.com)

Another site that used to be the go-to for local products and services, Merchant Circle offers yet another local space to advertise your dental services.

MapQuest (http://www.mapquest.com)

MapQuest used to be the go-to map service before Google and Apple came along. Despite it dropping in popularity, the platform still holds authority in many respects.

You cannot claim the listing yourself on MapQuest, but the platform's customer support is top-notch. Once your request is received, any duplicates or incorrect listings will usually be fixed right away.

Claiming, adding, and editing your information on the above directories is a major step toward more prominent Google rankings. However, we encourage you to go even further if you hope to drive an even greater amount of prospects and patients your way

Dental Directories

People looking for a dentist may not head to Google first. Instead, they may try a dental directory.

These directories may also be linked to from insurance providers. Therefore, ensure that your business is listed consistently across all directories, just like you did on the platforms we just visited.

Some additional directories we recommend include:

- **Health grades** https://www.healthgrades.com/
- **RateMDs** https://www.ratemds.com/
- **Healthtap** https://www.healthtap.com/
- **Doctor-Oogle** https://www.doctor-oogle.com/
- **Dentists.com** http://dentists.com/
- **Everydentist** https://www.everydentist.com/
- **Wellness** http://www.wellness.com/
- **Opencare** https://www.opencare.com/
- **Mytime** https://www.mytime.com/

Local Directories

There are also some local directories that are dedicated to various cities around the country. Look for directories in your local town, county, or city. You should also get listed on sites like Prepky.com, Cityof.com, TripAdvisor, and Shopcity.com.

Photo Hosting Sites

Photo hosting sites are an excellent source to add citations and send a strong local signal to Google. Some of the photo sites we recommend include the following.

- Pinterest for business
- Flickr
- Mobypicture
- Fotothing
- Instagram
- Fotolo

Step 4: External Link Building

By getting authoritative websites to link back to yours, you can get a nice Google boost. Remember, you have to be strategic about this, as buying links is frowned upon and can get you downgraded or banned outright by Google.

Instead, you will want to be ethical with your link building by following these steps.

- Anytime you host an event, such as a charity walk, get the website to link back to your dental practice.
- Ask your college to add your citation to their website as an alumnus.
- Make sure your website is listed on the CareCredit website.
- If you accept American Express, there is an option to get your business listed on their incredibly popular website.
- Get your site listed on Healthgrades and other dental directories so that patients asking questions can always find you.

Step 5: Turn-by-Turn Directions

Google Maps can help your practice get found when people use that app on their phones, but some people still use GPS devices like Garmin. To ensure you always get found by people looking for directions to your door, list your business on sites like Open Street, Here.com, and Map Share Tool.

Now that your office is optimized for a local audience, new leads looking for a dental practice should be able to find you. No matter if they take to Google or one of the dozens of local directories around the web, your practice will show up ready to be clicked-on and called.

Prospects stumbling upon your Google or Yelp or YellowPages profiles will be greeted by quality photos of your office, smiling faces of your staff, and all the information they need to make a positive buying decision.

Ideally, prospects will also be able to book an appointment right from whatever platform they happen to be visiting. That's the power of Local SEO, and the above steps are a must for any dental professional looking to succeed in today's digital-centric age.

CHAPTER 10: STAYING UP-TO-DATE WITH GOOGLE

Google will continue to make changes to how it displays search results in an effort to deliver premium content to its users. After all, Google is the most popular search engine used today, with millions of people relying on the platform each and every day.

As technology—and the way we use it—continues to evolve, so will the algorithms Google employs to satisfy its userbase. By staying up-to-date with Google's constant updates, your dental practice will remain visible to the quality patients searching for You.

Whether you work with a marketing company or choose the do-it-yourself approach, ensure your practice is taking advantage of the latest cutting-edge strategies—and efficiently implementing them—before the competition has a chance to catch up.

What follows are a few of the Google updates that have sent shockwaves through the digital marketing industry. Even though these tweaks have already happened, they completely changed the game, so it's important that you know about them.

By learning about these changes now, you will know the reasons *why* we use the techniques we do, and you'll remain ahead of the game so you never, ever fall behind. After all, knowledge is power, particularly when it comes to digital marketing.

Google Update #1: The Importance of Google Reviews

Google knows how much people trust reviews when it comes to making a buying decision. A raving review with five gold stars represents immediate social proof that your business is delivering first-rate dentistry that patients can trust.

Online reviews have been driving sales for years. Two examples include TripAdvisor and Amazon. Travelers head to TripAdvisor before planning a vacation to read real-life accounts of hotels, restaurants, and tour operators.

And before consumers make a purchase on Amazon, they read the reviews written by other buyers to see if the quality of the product is good and if consumers are largely satisfied post-sale.

The bottom line is that reviews help people avoid buyer's remorse. By only choosing the top-rated items and five-star trip options, consumers can spend their money wisely while being mostly assured a positive experience.

To help search users make better buying decisions, Google has now made it even easier to search through reviews before making a purchase. Take a look at the search below for "dentures in Austin, Texas."

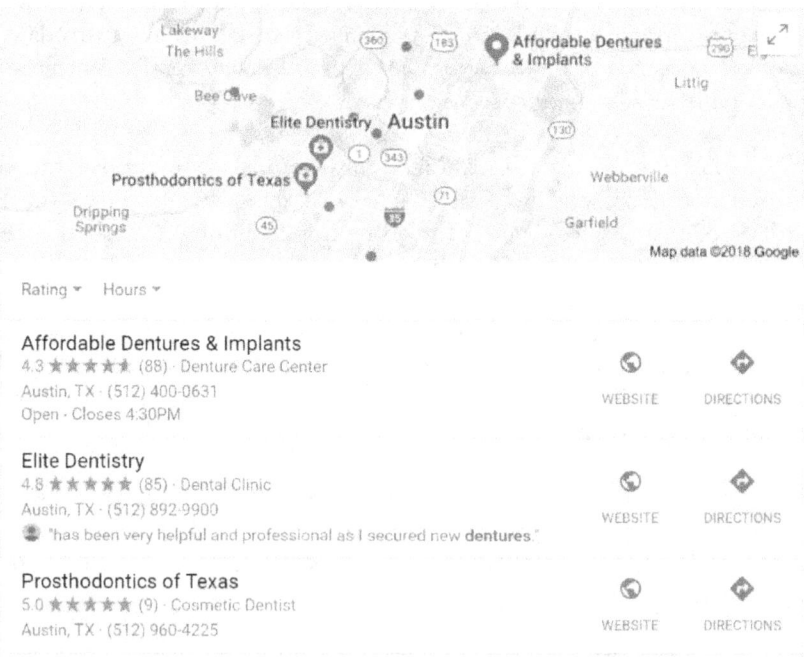

Google has now made it incredibly easy for people to select the best and closest dental office to them. The SERP offers a detailed map of the area along with pins so that you can determine which office is closest, but the SERP now offers something that wasn't there previously.

Google now offers the reviews and ratings of those office right beside the listings, helping the most popular office stand out and get noticed.

Google prioritizes which businesses will show up in local search results based on a review score. The higher and more frequent your Google reviews, the higher your Google ranking will be.

If your office doesn't have very many five-star reviews, this news may distress you. However, you must keep in mind that Google has a vested interest in providing the best experience for its users. Therefore, it makes sense that the search results would display the dental offices that are most raved about by its patients higher than the others.

Using the Google Maps app, users can also filter your reviews by their star rating. That way, a prospect can search for only those offices with four and five-star ratings, for example.

What does all this mean? It means that if you get a few one and two-star reviews, you unfortunately won't be able to hide them. Everyday users are becoming savvier to Google's customizable features daily, and filtering reviews helps people avoid bad experiences.

On the other hand, ask yourself this: Why would a patient choose a practice with all three-star reviews if they could get the same treatment from a dentist with all fives?

We are confident that you are already delivering five-star services to your patients. Now we only have to get your patients motivated to leave their own reviews on Google immediately following their appointments.

Many dentists make the mistake of only collecting reviews on third-party platforms like ZocDoc or 1800Dentist. Since we already know that patients start their search for a dental office on Google—and that Google is placing a lot of importance on the role reviews in its search results—it follows that Google is where you should be investing your time and effort when gathering online reviews.

Google Update #2: More Space for Google Ads

Compared to years past, you will now find that when you search on Google, the local map has been moved lower on the search results page, mostly to make room for more Google paid ads.

While this move is excellent for Google, it's also good news for your dental office, particularly if you use AdWords. Now, when you invest in Google Ads, your practice will have an increased opportunity to be seen by targeted, quality patients.

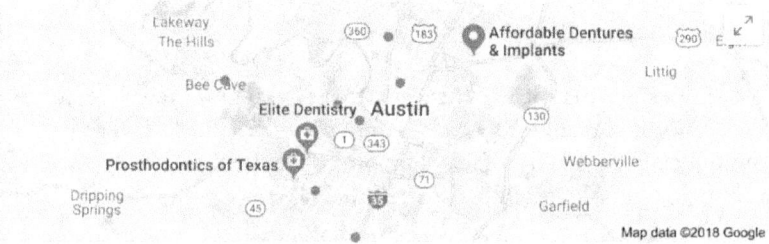

Google Update #3: Keyword Targeting

Earlier, we explained that long-tail keywords (groups of words or phrases) work best when optimizing for Google. That is because few people are typing "dentist" into the search box. Rather, patients are searching for the exact service and location they need.

Searching "emergency dentist in Portland, Oregon," for instance, is going to bring up much more specific and relevant results as opposed to simply searching "dentist."

Clearly, using long-tail keywords makes the most sense for your dental practice if you want to be found by patients who are desperately seeking your services. The good news is that Google is continuing to increase its focus on the importance of long-tail keywords, as well as the meaning behind the words.

When creating content for your digital marketing campaign, the long-tail keywords you use should coincide with what your patients want and need to know.

Those keywords should include the specific neighborhood or local subsection of the city where you are located, as well as the exact services your patients might be seeking. Use these long-tail keywords throughout your content where they naturally make sense. You don't want to "stuff" your website with phrases and keywords. If you focus on providing a fantastic experience for the patient, Google will continue to reward your practice now and in the future.

CHAPTER 11: GET ON FACEBOOK

Social media is one of those rare forms of marketing that enables you to reach out and connect with your prospects and patients wherever they happen to be, and on any device.

With smartphones in most pockets, tablet computers in many homes, and desktops and laptops in nearly every home and office, more people are connected to the web than ever before. And most web users are on at least one social network. Namely, Facebook.

Here is another area where our advice has diverged from years' past. We used to recommend that our clients create profiles on Google+, Twitter, and Facebook, in that order. Back then, that was the social network hierarchy.

Today, Facebook is king, and just about everyone visits the platform daily, sometimes multiple times per day, from teens to grandparents and all ages in between.

According to a report published by wearesocial.com, Facebook accounted for the majority of total social media user growth in 2016. Today, there are nearly two-billion daily users, which is more than any other social network.

What's great about Facebook is that the entire platform is populated by your friends and family. Therefore, when someone recommends a local business, you tend to respect their opinion, and pay attention.

It's the same with dental marketing. If someone gives your dental office a stellar review on Facebook, that review can potentially be seen by that person's friends, family, co-workers, and acquaintances, which means it can carry a lot of weight.

Statistics show that most people will buy a product or service based on a recommendation from a friend, and that's why Facebook should be a major aspect of your digital marketing campaign.

With only one social network to worry about, you won't find yourself spreading yourself too thin, and you will have at your disposal one of the most powerful marketing platforms in existence.

Engage with Existing Patients

Unfortunately, and in our experience, Facebook is not ideal for finding new patients. That's where Google reigns supreme. Everyone's favorite social platform can help spread the word about your practice, but it's typically not where patients begin their search for a dentist.

Facebook is excellent for sharing fun images to your Facebook account and can get your patients excited about their appointments, but Facebook marketing tends to be more about retention than acquisition.

Even if someone sees stellar reviews about your office on Facebook, they will still visit Google, in most cases, before they commit.

Therefore, the true value of Facebook marketing is your ability to authentically engaging with your current patients while building strong relationships that foster loyalty. That is what will keep patients coming back to your office for life.

The key to successful Facebook marketing is to share valuable and interesting content your audience cares about. Whatever you do, try not to contribute to the junk and noise flooding most people's newsfeeds. In other words, post only when you have something to post, and you'll retain your audience for years.

Give Your Social Media a Personalized Touch

Many dental offices that use social media hire a marketing company to manage their profiles, which – in our opinion – is a mistake. A marketing company won't understand what makes your practice unique. Third-party marketers also won't be able to share photos of your staff or add to discussions about what is happening in your neighborhood. Instead, the marketing company will likely fill your social media platforms with spammy content that receives little to no engagement because it is not coming from a place of authenticity.

That is why, while you should leave SEO and all the technical stuff to the experts, Facebook marketing is one area where you or your staff can offer significant value by taking the reins.

Our newsfeeds are already overflowing with so much garbage that we have become used to ignoring most of what we see. If your patients are not interested and engaged with your social media content, then you will fail to see any return on your investment. That's too much wasted time and money to even consider.

If you are going to use Facebook for marketing, you would do well to focus on humanizing and personalizing your profile and activity. Aim for real and authentic conversations between your dental office and the consumer.

Here are a few examples of excellent content to share with your Facebook followers:

- **Photos from holiday parties:** Patients will enjoy seeing their professional dentist and staff letting their hair down after hours. Don't go crazy but do be authentic for added effect.
- **FAQ videos with the dentist:** Doctors are busy people and don't have time to answer every question from every patient. A single video recorded and uploaded to Facebook can help patients become familiar with their dentist while getting their questions answered right from the source.
- **Special offers and discounts:** Patients will be more likely to take action on their decision to see a dentist if there are savings involved.
- **News and stories from your community:** Keeping your audience current on local events shows that you have their back, and they might return the favor by booking an appointment.
- **Featured smile makeovers from real-life patients:** Seeing a twisted smile become magazine-worthy may spur-on the patient who has been putting off Invisalign or braces.

Facebook may not be the best for attracting new patients, but the network is an excellent way to build meaningful relationships with consumers—provided you are willing to give it the necessary time and attention your followers deserve.

Now, let's get started setting up your Facebook account.

Step 1: Set Up a Facebook Account

To create your Facebook profile, visit www.Facebook.com and select the link near the bottom of the page that reads "Create a page for a celebrity, band, or business."

If you already have a personal Facebook account, click on the gear icon near the top right corner and select Create a Page. This is known as a fan page, which comes in a variety of styles.

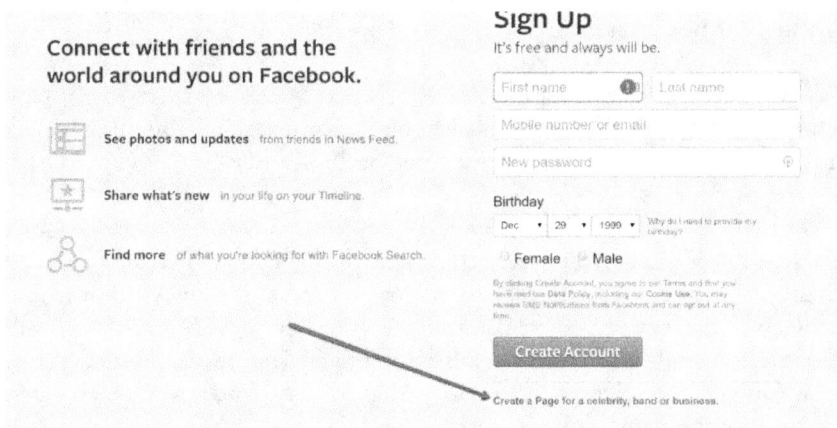

To create a fan page for a dental office, select the option "Local Business or Place."

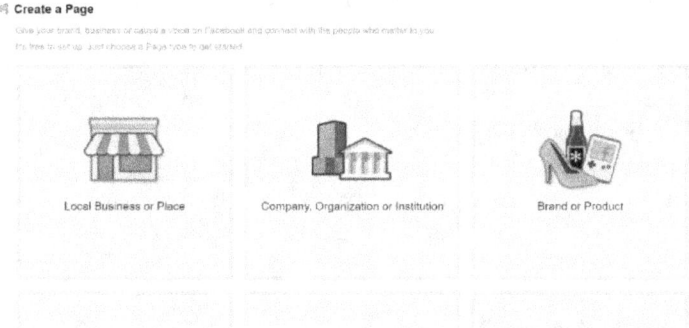

If you already have a Facebook account and you are not logged in, you will be asked to choose your category. We recommend that you select "Doctor."

Fill out the rest of the information, agree to the terms, and click the "Get

Started" button to begin developing your first Facebook marketing campaign.

Next, find the "About" tab in the left navigation pane. This is where you will describe your practice and what sets you apart from all the others in town.

Upload a photo from your computer or hotlink an image from somewhere online, such as your website, that accurately represents your practice and philosophy, such as a group photo featuring doctor and enthusiastic staff. The image you choose should be of the highest quality to put forth your best first impression.

When selecting your categories, list terms that Facebook users might type into the search box to find services like yours. For example, you might select Dentist, Root Canals, Teeth Extractions or Full-Smile Makeovers. These terms are, of course, your keywords.

Facebook will help you select the most popular keywords to use. The moment you begin to type, Facebook will try to predict the keyword by listing some viable alternatives. For example, if you type "tee," Facebook will automatically return the result "teeth whitening." Use these predictions to your advantage by selecting categories that will expand your reach even further across the Facebook network.

Your Story should be a concise summary of your About Us web page. Describe your office, philosophy, mission statement, doctors, and staff, and use a call-to-action to invite profile visitors to your website.

Your Facebook Admin Panel is where you can create new posts, upload photos, see who has "Liked" your page (a Like is a conversion in Facebook), and determine how your page is performing overall.

For right now, just make sure that your photos look good, your information is accurate, and that your posts are valuable, consistent, and constant for best results.

Six Facebook Marketing Steps

Yep, that's all it takes to get started marketing on Facebook! Here are six steps to keep your profile engaging, up-to-date, and converting.

Appoint A Social Media Ambassador

Facebook is one of those areas where too many cooks can spoil the soup. Facebook marketing works best when there is a consistent voice posting and responding to comments. When you have multiple people running the account, your followers will be faced with a hodgepodge of personalities that will make it difficult to know which one to get comfortable with.

For best results, recruit a Facebook marketer from within your ranks. That person will oversee posting, curating posts from other dental professionals, responding to comments, and keeping up with the campaign's progress.

This is not job that can be done every now and again. Facebook should be updated often, at least four times per week. Ideally, your Facebook marketer will take photos and videos from within the office for added authenticity.

Select someone who is sociable and enthusiastic and who loves using Facebook on their own time. While they may be tempted to use Facebook for personal uses during business hours, you can bet a savvy Facebook user will be able to hit the ground running without much training.

Make Inviting Friends Fun

Just because you have one person running your Facebook campaign doesn't mean the other staff can't get involved. The entire office should invite their friends and family to like and share the office Facebook page.

You can even generate excitement among your staff and patients alike by hosting a contest to see who can recommend the most Facebook fans to your page. The winner can receive a $25 gift card to a local eatery, or something of similar value.

Generate Excitement

Facebook is one of those platforms you check when you're bored or standing in line somewhere or at home parked in front of the TV. It's used by all sorts of people in all types of circumstances, but all of us who use Facebook have one thing in common: We want to see something interesting.

Telling your Facebook marketer to be interesting is one thing, but it's quite another to actually be that way. To be interesting on Facebook, it helps to pay attention to what your competitors are posting. Most likely, they are posting friendly pics from inside the office, humorous dental themed content, and thought-provoking dentistry news.

Don't keep your competitor research to your area. Search for dental fan pages from Miami, Phoenix, Chicago, and other mass markets that sport higher competition. You can even borrow or "curate" that content for use on your own page. As long as it fits your target market, there is no limit to the amount or type of content you can post to your Facebook page.

Engage People

While you are searching for posts to curate, begin to pay attention to the comments on those posts. Facebook is terrific in that it allows you to "listen in" on the conversations your prospects and patients are having. You can even jump in and be helpful when you can!

Specials and Promotions

The next time you offer free teeth whitening, a discounted oral health exam, or free Invisalign consultation, let your patients know by posting to your Facebook fan page. You never know when you might entice someone to call, email or come in to take you up on your special offer.

Be Visual

The words accompanying your posts are important, but Facebook is largely a visual platform. Therefore, you will want to use your best office photos that successfully promote your dental office, products, and services.

Studies show that Facebook posts that include photos receive 120-times more engagement than posts with mere text. For best results, post photographs of smiling staff and patients.

Finding Fresh Content to Post

Go Behind-the-Scenes

Showing what goes on in the areas patients aren't usually exposed to is an excellent way to make your dental practice seem more "human." This, in turn, helps to build strong relationships with prospective and current patients.

Smiling and Impromptu Staff Photos

Facebook is an excellent way to endear patients to your staff, the very professionals who will be caring for their teeth.

When sharing photographs, use the best equipment and bright lighting. The images should be clear, adequately sized, and positive in nature. Done well, and Facebook can be an outward projection of your staff's bubbly personality.

Make Videos and Occasionally Go Live

Videos, especially live videos, are also a great way to show what goes on in non-patient areas. Try and keep videos between one-minute and a minute-twenty in length. Videos can be of staff and patients. Used properly, and videos can help to capture the authentic interactions you engage in daily while entertaining, inspiring, delighting, and educating.

Videos can also help to make patients feel more comfortable by highlighting patient fears, employee humor, success stories, and dental tips.

Community Work

Your fans will love to hear about your philanthropic efforts, so don't bypass any opportunity to capture and post about volunteering or donating funds or time to charitable causes in your community through the use of photos or video.

Contests and Promotions

Encouraging followers to compete is one of the best ways to get people to pay attention to your profile, and can be excellent for lead generation. Contests and Promotions have a viral quality about them and are fundamental to the growth of your page.

A Contest can be something as simple as giving away free movie tickets to the latest blockbuster. To enter, users must leave a Facebook review or post about the dental office somehow.

Promotions can be advertised the same way. You can even turn your promotion into a contest by giving a prize to the person who draws enough attention to your special offer.

Putting It All Together

Facebook marketing should include a healthy mix of informative posts, behind the scenes pictures, as well as staff and patient photos and video. If you find that one particular post is shared, and liked, more than most, pay attention and do your best to find out why. That way, you replicate your stellar results in the future.

Typically, any post including a photo of your staff will do better than a generic photo of a disembodied smiling mouth, for example. Try to be creative and combine multiple elements, such smiling faces and new technology, or happy patients and a video of the doctor discussing a frequently asked question.

Another example is to share useful information about brushing while including a photo of the dentist in the post. This gives the effect of making it seem as though the dentist is making the statement, lending the post far more credibility.

Transparency Only

Facebook users have little tolerance for fake or unauthentic posts. If it's not authentic, then don't even bother posting it. Never post to Facebook just to post. Your content should always have a purpose or reason.

Organizing and Managing Your Facebook Marketing Campaign

It is best to have a plan in mind before you begin posting to your fan page. For Example, you might decide to create four posts per week that consist of the following topics.

- **Special Offer:** Free Invisalign consultation
- **Success Story:** A patient had his braces off and is going off to college with extreme confidence!
- **Highlight a Staff Member:** Dental Hygienist Mary got engaged and is planning for a wedding in May!
- **A Point of Local Interest or Funny Meme:** A PSA photo from a Miami dental office depicting a patient with a hurt tooth that says, "I knew I should've used that bottle opener."

When developing your plan, pinpoint the days you will post, such as every Monday, Tuesday, Wednesday, and Thursday, and schedule your posts a few weeks in advance, if possible.

Posting with a consistent schedule while knowing what you want to post beforehand can make Facebook marketing easy to schedule and maintain.

The above example schedule also gives you a good combination of posts so you're always switching things up.

You can also use a tool like Buffer (https://buffer.com/) that allows you to schedule Facebook posts in advance. Then, you will only have to worry about responding to any comments or questions that show up as a result of your posting strategy.

It is extremely important to engage with your audience. Earlier we gave you tips on how to respond to Facebook comments. Use that advice to keep a positive dialog going with your audience that culminates in a dental appointment.

Facebook marketing is not something you can set and forget. When a comment or question comes in, respond as quickly as possible.

Finally, don't forget to ask for shares. After all, if you don't ask for shares, you won't give your audience any incentive to spread the word far and wide about your dental practice.

Get a Facebook page your prospects and patients will love. Download the ultimate Facebook marketing guide FREE at http://www.firegang.com/book-bonuses/

CHAPTER 12: REPUTATION MANAGEMENT AND ONLINE REVIEWS

You can contribute to a stellar reputation by providing excellent products and services, treating your patients with respect, and making sure your office and dental environment are clean and organized.

While your offline reputation is carried along by word-of-mouth, your online reputation is largely centered around Internet-based reviews. We recently covered Google reviews and you saw how prominent reviews are in the SERPs.

Facebook also uses reviews to help users make intelligent buying decisions. So does Amazon, TripAdvisor, and dozens of others.

While you should always focus on sending your satisfied patients to Google first to leave a review, Facebook should be a close second.

Google reviews are posted by real people, but Facebook reviews have added legitimacy. That is because anyone can create a Google account, but Facebook accounts are usually authenticated and friended by the person's closest relatives and associates.

By populating Facebook with positive reviews about your practice, you will add irrefutable social proof that your office is valuable and trustworthy.

Not only that, but – just like in Google - more positive reviews can help you appear more frequently and prominently in Facebook search results.

When it comes to reviews, either on Google or Facebook, make sure you are constantly generating more.

The fact is, four five-star reviews from three years ago just won't cut it. Your online reviews need to be current. That is, you need to ask every satisfied patient for them.

People reading your Google reviews will notice if most are from months or years ago. Five-star reviews from this month, however, can be very convincing for new patients in search of a dentist.

The Psychology of Reviews

As humans, we put a lot of weight into other people's experiences. In a way, we try to predict our own experience based on the experiences of others.

Take online reviews, for example. If you can convince your prospective patients that loads of locals have used your services and remained satisfied, you have a much greater chance of luring those individuals into your office.

FIREGANG FACT: It's said that 89% of Internet users trust online reviews as much as a personal recommendation.

Here are some other facts about reviews that may interest you.

> **More than 70% of Americans read online reviews before making a purchase.**

> **Around 63 percent of consumers are more likely to purchase from a site if it has ratings and reviews.**

> **If your dental office doesn't have any online reviews, you could be sending away 60-70% of your prospective patients.**

Even having very few reviews can be damaging to your offline reputation. A practice with two or three reviews looks small and insignificant, especially when compared to a dental office with dozens of five-star reviews.

Even if those three reviews are incredibly boastful, patients would rather trust the experiences of many than the opinions of a few.

For this reason, more often than not, it is the doctors with the most positive online reviews that collect the most new patients in any given area.

How Many Reviews Do You Need?

Society makes decisions based largely on reviews. We trust the cumulative reviews of the masses more than a single review from a friend.

The friend giving the recommendation may be undereducated in this area or easily satisfied, after all. Or maybe the friend is too polite to tell it like it is. Or maybe the friend did have an excellent experience, but is that typical of this particular office?

There are too many variables to trust a single review, even if the viewpoints originate from someone we dearly trust!

There is a direct correlation between reviews and new patients. Since day one, we have been pushing clients to gather more online reviews. But still, clients resisted. More often than not, if there is one area where clients tend to slack off, it's the act of gathering online reviews on a consistent basis.

It's not that clients don't want more online reviews. Many fear learning what the public really thinks about them. However, this is one of those difficult things that must be committed to if you desire to be successful.

How many reviews do you need? We recommend you collect at least ten new reviews each month. Kept in perpetuity, all those reviews will soon add up to tons of new business.

Put simply, more reviews separate the good dentists from the bad. And for you to get more reviews, it is a good idea to collaborate and partner with your marketing company.

How to Gather More Online Reviews

Your job is to make it very easy for current patients to leave their opinions and deepest inner thoughts about your office. The first step is so easy, anyone can do it.

Ask for Them

How do you get people to leave reviews? Simple. You just ask. You don't need to give them a comment card or point them to a link. Just tell them to go on Google and leave a review. They'll usually take care of the rest themselves.

Again, we recommend you send your satisfied patients to Google to leave reviews first, then Facebook, then the other platforms if need be.

The bottom line is that you are unlikely to get online reviews unless you ask for them, and yet reviews are such a make or break element of a digital marketing campaign. If you don't gather constant online reviews, your Google rankings will suffer, and potential new patients will choose another office with a higher review rating.

The entire office should work together if you hope to maximize the amount of reviews your office receives. While everyone is encouraged to ask for reviews, you should never ask for "positive" reviews specifically.

Asking for positive reviews gives off a negative vibe, and – let's be honest: Are you really going to convinece someone to rave about your office if they recently had a bad time?

People are going to leave their thoughts, and relay their experiences as they see them in their mind's eye.

Your staff can restrict the asking to only those who have enjoyed a positive experience, but your staff should definitely learn *why* reviews are important, and what's at risk by not asking for them.

For best results, give your staff goals and incentives to work toward. The more they want it, the more reviews your practice will collect, and the more patients you'll attract.

Review Software

Perpetually collecting a large volume of new reviews can be time-consuming and sometimes impossible for a busy dental office. To help, we employ a variety of applications that put the review gathering process on autopilot.

Podium, for example, makes it easy for people to leave reviews by texting or emailing a link. That way, patients can leave reviews at home, work, or on the go with their computers and mobile devices.

One of our clients, Gastonia Family Dentistry, uses Podium. The staff members have iPads and go through how to leave a review with each patient following their appointments.

Does this system work? It must. Gastonia Family Dentistry has over 700 reviews drawing new patients into their office.

Create a Review Us Page

You can encourage loads more online reviews by creating a new page on your website dedicated to online reviews. The page you create will consist of nothing more than icons from today's top review sites like Google and Facebook along with buttons that contain strong calls-to-action like, "Review Us!"

Once that page is completed, tell all of your current patients about it. You can do this before their appointments as they are checking in, during their appointments, or as they are settling their accounts prior to leaving.

Video Reviews

Nothing is more powerful for attracting new patients than a review straight from the source's mouth. Video reviews are pure gold but are often overlooked because of the amount of work involved. This is a huge mistake. Remember, it's that extra effort that sets your dental practice apart.

Why Video Reviews Work

More Authentic

Video reviews are perceived as more authentic than written reviews. They allow people to put a face and name to who the patients are, instead of reading text that could have been written by anyone. This tangibility not only lends the videos more credibility, but it also fosters a relationship between patient and practice.

Establish Trust

Video reviews allow potential patients to observe whether the filmed patient's interests and backgrounds resemble their own, establishing trust between the reviewer and the audience. Patients can see the results of various dental procedures in real life, making it easier to imagine those procedures being done on them. The more people learn about your office and services, the more personally connected they will feel, and the more likely they will be to schedule an appointment.

Emotional Connection

Video reviews also provide you with the perfect opportunity to showcase your staff's personalities and office atmosphere, so customers feel more connected to your practice.

Be sure to film several videos, not just one. Remember that each video increases the amount of time viewers spend on your website, which is a strong indication to Google of your site's authority.

Emotional Investment

You will always want to guide the interaction while filming the video. Don't let the patient ramble or go off script. The best way to guide the video is to ask plenty of questions.

When asking questions, entice the patient to discuss their concerns, issues, and the challenges they faced. Don't forget to ask about their motivation for getting the procedure done in the first place.

Most of all, when recording a video review, encourage the patient to talk on an emotional level. Here are some questions to ask to spark emotional investment.

> **How did the state of your previous smile affect your confidence?**

> **How much has your confidence improved since the procedure?**

> **Would you recommend this service to others?**

A good video review doesn't just take the audience on the journey; It gets them emotionally invested in the outcome.

Use Positive Reviews to Their Maximum Advantage

The moment a positive review comes in, you should respond to it. Thank patients for leaving their thoughts and tell them that you can't wait to see them back in your office.

Patient engagement is powerful. Responding to reviews shows your audience that you care about your patients, and that you have a strong desire to continually improve your services. Responding may encourage others to leave their thoughts, as well, when they otherwise may have passed on the opportunity.

Never give a patient an incentive to leave a review. Not only is it poor ethics, but it's also against FTC rules. If you are caught giving money, goods, or services in exchange for reviews, you can be fined big-time.

Instead, gather reviews the legal, ethical, and organic way. Provide excellent service, then ask your patients for reviews in person, using software, or via any other means.

Three Rules for Responding to Reviews

Something we can't stress enough here at Firegang is for our clients to proactively respond to all user reviews, particularly the not-so-positive ones. The magic formula for responding to reviews is to, first and foremost, acknowledge and answer the patient's questions. You should also offer useful suggestions and - most importantly - provide a contact email address at the end of the post.

If you are worried about responding to online reviews out of fear of revealing personal information or violating HIPAA and any local/state privacy laws, here are the three rules for responding to reviews that you are encouraged to follow.

1. **Never discuss patient names or personal details publicly unless you have received written permission from your patients to do so.**

2. **Be general when giving advice about the overall well-being and care of your patients' oral health. Think long and hard about how to respond before you commit. Once your response is live, there is no going back.**

3. **Take the situation offline by telling the patient that you would love to discuss the matter in private, then leave your phone number.**

Mitigate the Damage of Online Reviews

Ideally, patients would leave nothing but five-star reviews that prove that you're the best dental professional in town. However, even the best dentists have received at least one less-than-stellar review.

The good news is that people reading reviews can be quite forgiving. They are also intelligent and can determine that a single one-star review among a sea of five-stars means nothing in the grand scheme.

Maybe that one-star reviewer had a bad day, the person reading the review might think.

Therefore, most patients won't mind if your practice receives one or two bad reviews.

In fact, owning nothing but five-star reviews can make your office look shady. For all anyone knows, your staff wrote them all. Therefore, refrain from trying to hide negative reviews and certainly don't write any yourself.

Instead, accept your negative reviews as a way to project an honest, credible, and authentic image of your dental practice. As counterintuitive as it seems, prospective patients are more likely to believe your positive reviews when they know that one, or a few, negative reviews exist.

If and when you do get a negative review, follow these six steps to mitigate any damage to your online reputation.

Respond Quickly

The moment a negative review comes in, forget about the potential 30 patients you might lose and take time to respond to the one person who left the review in the first place.

Be Brief

If you respond to the review with more than two sentences, you can come across as being defensive. For best results, keep your response quick and to the point.

Be Empathetic

Let the reviewer know that you know exactly what he or she is going through and that you want nothing more than to ensure their satisfaction. Get a dialog started and find out what is truly bothering them. For good measure, make sure you thank the person for leaving the review.

Offer Something of Value

Gauge what you feel the reviewer most wants and then seek to provide it, either in the form of a free offer, discount, or complete refund. The small amount of money you lose turning a negative comment into a positive one could earn your practice thousands more later on.

Know When to Say When

Do not get into a heated debate with a patient online, especially if the person leaving the negative review resorts to ad hominem attacks or starts making impossible demands, such as urging you to fire of one of your staff members.

To handle situations like these, tell the reviewer that you are sorry about their dissatisfaction; that you will do whatever it takes to make it right; and then ask to speak to the person in private. Leave your phone number and then leave it alone.

Use Negativity to Improve

It is best to discuss negative reviews with your staff during regular business meetings. Decide what comments are truthful and what can be improved upon. Then, use that information to make your practice and the staff who run it even better.

A Takeaway From Online Reviews

Instead, of having every patient leave generic, positive feedback, you should encourage an open and honest dialog without fear of permanently damaging your online reputation.

Using review management software such as Podium can keep your staff processes organized and will ensure you get more reviews for your digital campaign.

Now it is time to discuss the very best way to dominate the local SERPs that doesn't involve organic search engine optimization. We are talking about paid search advertising. With the proper budget and the following advice, your ads will show up for relevant users anytime they search for your keywords. Your job is to entice them to click-through your ads so that they'll call, email, or come in for a visit.

CHAPTER 13: PAY-PER-CLICK SEARCH ENGINE ADVERTISING

In this section, we are going to cover both Google and Facebook paid advertising. Those are only two platforms in a club of thousands, but you should focus your time and attention on Google, first, and Facebook, second, to maximize your success.

How to Advertise on Google

Google has a robust and popular advertising platform called AdWords. Paid search ads are the Google listings that accompany the organic listings on the top and bottom portions of the SERPs whenever you search for, "dentist in Austin," for example.

The type of paid advertising we'll be discussing is known as PPC marketing or pay-per-click. This is the type of advertising that Google uses to monetize its search engine and is incredibly effective at putting any type of business in front of viable prospects.

By developing the Google AdWords platform, the search giant attempted to "level the playing field," allowing anyone to get on the first page of Google, as long as they had the expertise and budget.

The premise was simple: As long as advertisers used relevant keyword terms and created quality ads over time, Google would reward them with top-billing listings.

Each AdWords user gets a "Quality Score," which affects "AdRank," which means that advertisers who heed Google's rules will typically always come out ahead.

This means that AdWords can help you rank prominently on Google quickly, as long as you have the skills, know-how, proper budget, and time to garner a stellar reputation.

One thing's for sure. By monetizing search with the PPC model, Google has become one of the wealthiest and most successful companies in the history of the world.

To get a better understanding of the AdWords platform, let's explore how the advertising model works at its core.

Google AdWords

Before you get started with AdWords, it is important for you to understand that spending money on PPC does not guarantee results or that your ads will show up for relevant searches 100% of the time.

When a search user enters one of your keywords into their Google search box, AdWords will rank ads based on two factors: quality score and maximum bid. That's where the expertise and budget come into play.

We've somewhat covered quality score. The better your ads are over time – in that they adhere to Google's requirements for quality ads – the higher your quality score.

The score is a number from 1 to 10 that takes into account your ads, landing pages (the pages that prospects will land on by clicking your ads), and the keywords you use based on their relevancy to popular searches.

The higher your quality score and maximum bid, the more likely your ads will rank in the first three Google search positions. Your job is to create ads that are enticing and relevant so that prospects and patients are quick to click.

In creating this system, Google has made it so that the highest bid doesn't necessarily determine top rankings. An advertiser must strive to deliver the very best if he or she hopes to attain the top spots.

You will be charged a certain amount of your budget each time your ads are clicked. The amount you are charged depends on the competitiveness of the keyword in question. The more competitive the keyword, the more you will be charged.

This is why it is essential that you set a daily budget so that you don't drain your finances the very first day your ads are run. Once you reach your daily budget, your ads will disappear from the rotation for that day until the next day, when your ads and daily budget will appear all over again.

That is the AdWords PPC advertising model in a nutshell. In this section, we are going to show you how to set up an AdWords account and prepare your first campaign to go live. Don't worry, we'll explain all of the basic settings and preference choices, and we'll also touch on the more advanced options just in case you want to take your PPC performance to the next level.

A Word About Results

Many dental professionals come to us after failing at a self-run PPC campaign, and this only leaves them with a bad taste in their mouths.

If you have had a previously bad experience with PPC marketing, we ask that you give it one more shot using the steps we have outlined below. While immediate results are certainly possible, we ask that you give it at least three months to deliver the results you are hoping for.

Later in this section, we will teach you how to analyze and test various data points to further optimize your PPC campaign and enhance the results you experience.

We are providing you with this knowledge so that you can check your marketers' progress or DIY, if you choose to go that route.

However, we strongly caution against running a Google AdWords campaign while simultaneously attempting to run a busy dental office. Your ads require constant mentoring, testing, and tweaking to find the ad-and-landing-page combinations your audience most responds to.

AdWords is not a simple affair. If you get it wrong, you will deplete your budget quickly with few, if any, leads to show for it.

Hire experts and get AdWords right for a supercharged ad campaign that fills up your schedule.

Want an AdWords campaign that drives leads and puts patients in your chair? Call (800) 398-0979 or email sales-team@firegang.com. You can also visit https://www.firegang.com/ to learn more.

How to Create a Google AdWords Account

Visit the Google AdWords homepage (https://AdWords.google.com) and sign in using your Google account information. Next, answer the questions Google asks, such as which country you reside in, your time zone, and the currency you would like AdWords to use.

Once your account is confirmed, you will be ready to create your first AdWords campaign and ad group.

Proper Organization is the Key to AdWords Success

Structure your PPC account in order, from broader campaign ideas to more narrowed-down ad groups and keywords. This is known as campaign segmenting.

For example, you might segment your campaigns based on your products and treatments or your general location. You can segment your campaigns based on how well they perform, or how poorly, or how much you have set to bid for certain keywords.

The segment hierarchy you decide to use is completely up to you, but we recommend that you organize your account properly for best results. Proper organization will also allow for easier testing later on. We recommend creating another tab in your spreadsheet to keep track of all AdWords campaigns, ad groups, and keywords.

A sample ad campaign may seek to build awareness and drive conversions for dental implants. The campaign titled "Dental Implants" might then have ad groups that focus on partial implants, full implants, and implant dentures. You might then have another ad group titled "Teeth Whitening" with ad groups that focus on the various types of treatments, such as take-home teeth whitening kits and laser teeth whitening.

The ad groups you create can have an infinite number of ads; it all depends on the keywords you hope to optimize for and the budget you have available to make them run.

We recommend that you set three to five ad groups per campaign for easy maintenance. You can always create more, but we find this number to be the sweet spot, especially when you have multiple ad groups running simultaneously. And if your practice offers ten or more services, with three to five ad groups running per service, trust us, you will have more than your share to manage.

Whatever you do, don't become overwhelmed. We will show you how to easily maintain, optimize, and supercharge your PPC campaigns once they go live.

Creating Your First AdWords Campaign

To create your first campaign, click on the Campaigns tab near the top of the page and find the "Add Campaign" button.

When you click on that button, you will be asked to specify the network where you want your ads to be displayed. We recommend you select the option "Search Network."

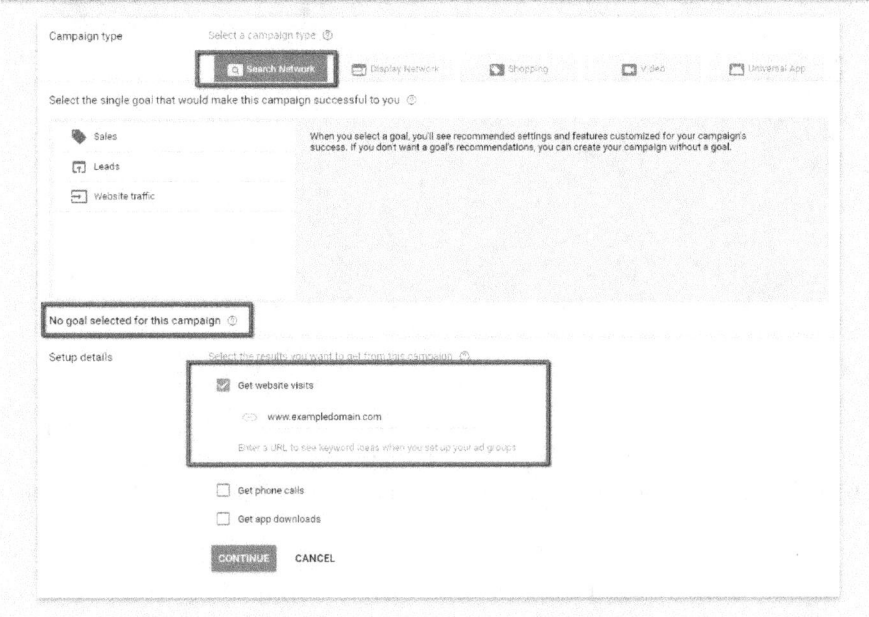

As Google suggests, this is the best opportunity to reach the most customers. The other options do have their merits, but for beginners (and until you can learn the intricacies of the AdWords mechanism), it is best to keep things simple in order to maximize the effectiveness of the ads you will create.

Ad Campaign Settings

Here you will be asked to name your first campaign. We recommend you select a product or service, such as tooth extractions. Keep the type of ad and the network settings in their default positions for now; you can always change these at a later date.

Devices

We recommend you keep the default setting for devices, which indicates that your ads will show up properly on all types of devices. Later, you will learn how to test your results to find out how your prospects and patients are finding and landing on your online presence. If you find that most of your visitors are using tablet computers to access your site, for example, you will want to come back to this setting in the future and select "Tablets" with "Full Browsers" when prompted.

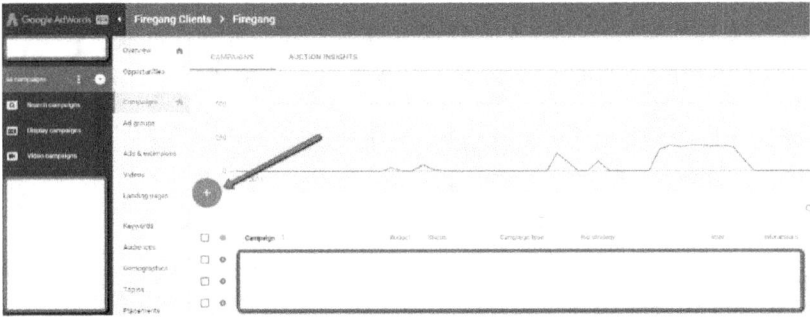

Locations

This is where you should set your local area since you rely on local customers first and foremost. Select the radio button "Let Me Choose" and enter all the geographic modifiers your audience might use to find your dental office.

On the other hand, if you are selling products through your website to a national or even worldwide audience, this is where you will alter the settings to reflect those changes. Then, select the languages you wish your ads to display.

Bid Strategy

This is where you will tell AdWords how you want to bid for the keywords you want to optimize for. We recommend that you keep the default setting, "I'll manually set my bids for clicks." This is where you will set a maximum cost-per-click (CPC) for each keyword in question. Your daily budget will never be charged over that amount for any single click.

The other option is to put AdWords in charge of your bids, which could turn out to be an outrageous amount, depending on the competitive nature of the keyword in question. For right now, set your own bids and reserve allowing AdWords to do it until you have gained more experience with the PPC advertising model.

Default Bid

This is the maximum bid amount you will be willing to pay for the first ad group in your campaign. We recommend that you set this amount low for now, such as $6, until you have more data to justify bidding higher amounts. You can always change this amount later.

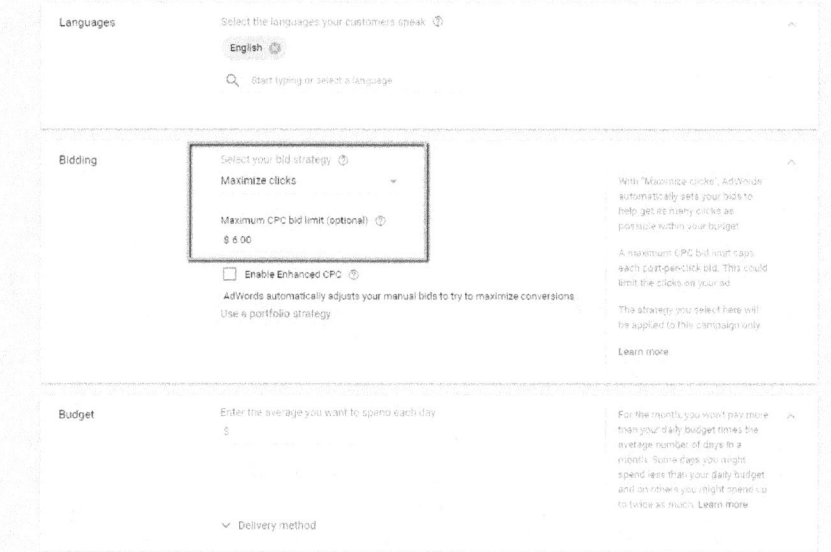

Daily Budget

This is the maximum amount you are willing to spend on your pay-per-click ads on any given day. For example, if your bid amount is $5 and your daily limit is $10, your ads can be clicked twice before they disappear from the network until the next day, whereby your daily budget will start all over again.

The minimum amount Google will allow per day is $10. We recommend that you divide your total budget by the number of days in the month so that you can maximize your click allowance and, as you will soon learn how to do, improve your ad conversions.

Ad Extensions

We recommend that you select all three ad extensions offered to you by AdWords. Doing so will allow you to display your office location, web addresses to specific pages on your site, and phone number directly in your ads. In theory, prospects who then see your ads won't even have to click through to your website in order to convert.

Creating Your First Ad Group

Set your Ad Group name, which should be a subset of your campaign category, such as "Veneers" under the campaign "Cosmetic Dentistry."
Now you are ready to create your ad.

Character Limits

You are allowed two headlines per ad and each one can only be 30 characters in length. Next, you get two display URL paths, which can only be 15 characters, and then you get 80 characters for the description.

With so little space allowed, it is wise to learn how to condense your ideas into just a few words or less.

Stand Apart

Take a look at a few of the ads your competitors have in active rotation. Simply search for your keywords and examine the ads that show up, their titles, and ad bodies. You can then click through to view the landing pages associated with those ads and use this research to make your AdWords ads even more effective.

Promotions, Prices, and Special Offers

Your ads will receive a higher number of conversions if you mention specific promotions, like free teeth cleaning; prices, like $25 off teeth whitening; and special offers, like refer a friend and get $25.

Benefits of Clicking Through

As concisely as possible and using the small space allotted, you must successfully explain to your audience exactly what they will get out of clicking through to the landing page you have set out for them to visit.

Use At Least One Keyword

Include a relevant keyword in your ad at least once, in the title, body, or both for best results. Don't include your keywords just to include them. They should merge naturally with the other words you have chosen.

Matching Landing Page

Don't just send leads to your home page. You will get far more conversions if you set a dedicated page that is relevant to the ad your prospects are expected to click. This could be your teeth whitening webpage or a stand-alone landing page designed simply to gather prospect information. A dedicated page will be easier to test, since the traffic will come solely from ad click-throughs and can be easily experimented with and tweaked to improve results.

Clear Calls-to-Action

As with all other CTAs, don't be afraid to tell your prospects exactly what you expect them to do. If you have done everything else correctly, your soon-to-be patients will gladly comply.

Heed the Rules

You can capitalize the first letters of each word, and you are encouraged to do so to increase conversions, but you should never capitalize every letter of any single word. Don't use excessive punctuation or repeat words for added emphasis, such as Free Free Free; and refrain from using numbers to represent words, such as Braces 4 Less.

Google will penalize you for breaking the rules, and this will affect your AdWords quality score. The higher your score, the lower you will pay for your ads overall. The lower your score, the more you will pay and the fewer conversions you will enjoy, making your PPC campaigns ineffective or, worse, useless.

Spend time learning about any recently updated rules so that you can avoid penalties or the feared Google ban-hammer, which will remove your account from the AdWords platform entirely.

Choose Your Ad Keywords

Here is where you will enter all of the keywords that you want your ads to show up for. You can enter one keyword per line. Choose relevant service keywords, geography keywords, and brand keywords, as well as any synonyms and related terms.

Google also provides a list of suggested keywords based on the name of your campaign and ad group. There is no limit to the number of keywords you can select, but the more you use, the higher the chances that your ads will show up for relevant search queries. We recommend including all of the relevant keywords on your list, as well as the ones Google suggests, for best results.

Choose a Few Negative Keywords

AdWords allows you to block searches that have nothing to do with your campaigns, ad groups, or keywords. The terms that you wish to block are known as negative keywords. An example might be someone who searches for "dental clinic in Tucson." You don't want your ads showing up for people looking for medical clinics, plastic surgery clinics, walk-in clinics, and so on.

You may not know which negative keywords to set right now. Later, you will learn how to analyze your AdWords and overall traffic data. You will also be able to determine what keyword terms search engine users are entering into their search boxes before they click on your ads. If you notice any terms that don't apply, enter them as negative keywords to prevent your ads from showing up for those terms in the future.

Complete the AdWords Billing Process

You will be asked to set up a credit card, debit card, or checking account to fund your Google AdWords account. You can pre-pay your account or you can opt to have Google remove the money from your account at various intervals. Generally speaking, Google will remove payment from your account monthly, unless you set up pre-paid service.

We recommend that you also keep an eye out for free AdWords coupons, which offer a discount on your first AdWords campaign. You will typically receive a coupon in the mail the moment you sign up, but we can't promise anything.

Expand Your AdWords Campaign

Once you have created your first ad group, continue to create ad groups and assign keywords for all of your other products and services that you want to optimize for. Once those are created and your billing system is established, your ads will go live. You can check the status of your ads any time by clicking the home tab at the top of the AdWords platform.

Home

Here you can view each of your campaigns, ad groups, and keywords, as well as how well or poorly they are performing. Right at the top of the page is a breakdown of the data for easy reference.

The horizontal bar near the top of the page shows the number of overall clicks your ads have generated, the impressions they have received (the number of times your ads have shown up on individual screens), the click-through rate percentage, the average cost-per-click amount, and the overall cost to your AdWords budget.

If you want to manage your campaigns, click on the menu tab of the same name to the right of the Home tab.

Campaigns

Here you will be able to create new campaigns or edit your current ones. You also get a quick snapshot of how each campaign is performing.

Opportunities

AdWords offers you suggestions on how to improve your AdWords campaigns based on the current data. When you first create your campaigns, ad groups, and keywords, the Opportunities page will merely explain the service and display a preview of things to come.

You will need to wait a while after your PPC campaigns go live to receive the platform's useful and practical advice. We recommend that you check back to the Opportunities tab often to keep up with your latest AdWords suggestions.

Tools

Change History

Here you can view the changes you have applied to your account, as well as edit your account history however you see fit.

Google Analytics

Google's proprietary web data-tracking platform seamlessly merges with AdWords to provide you with even more traffic and conversion data.

Google Merchant Center

This section is for product ads, which you would use if you selected Product Sales when you created your campaign.

Keyword Planner

We will cover this AdWords tool in the very next section. You will use it to further hone your keyword list and improve your organic and paid search engine optimization efforts.

Display Planner

For image or video ads, Display Ads under Tools will enable you to establish your settings.

Ad Preview and Diagnosis

Click on this tab to search for your ads just as you would in Google. The difference is that you won't be charged for ad impressions as you would if you searched normally. This allows you to check and alter your ads before or during their current rotation.

Conversions

This tab under Tools allows you to track the keywords that are receiving the most attention: click-throughs, downloads, calls, visits, or email forms.

Setting Up AdWords Conversion Tags

You can set up an AdWords conversion tracking tag directly from AdWords. To set this up, you will need to supply the required AdWords Conversion ID and Conversion Label, an optional Conversion Value, Order ID, and Currency Code.

First, select Conversions by clicking on the wrench icon.

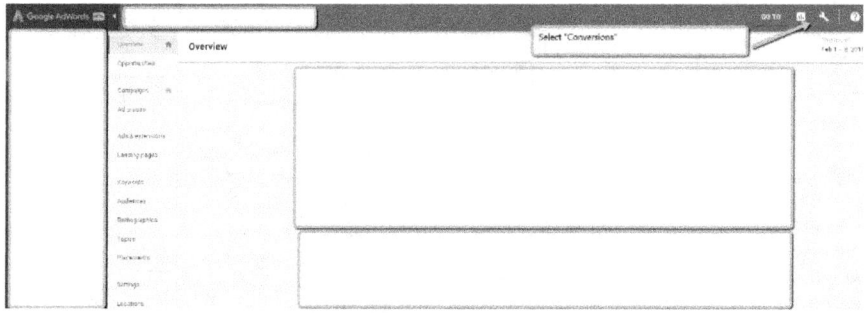

Then, click the + button to add a Conversion Action.

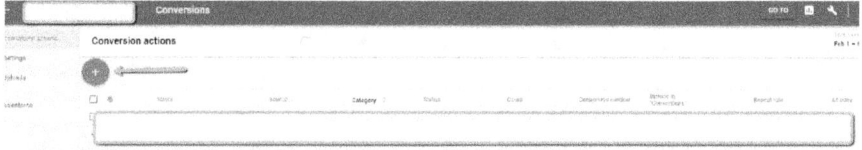

On the next screen, select the option "Track sales and other actions on your website."

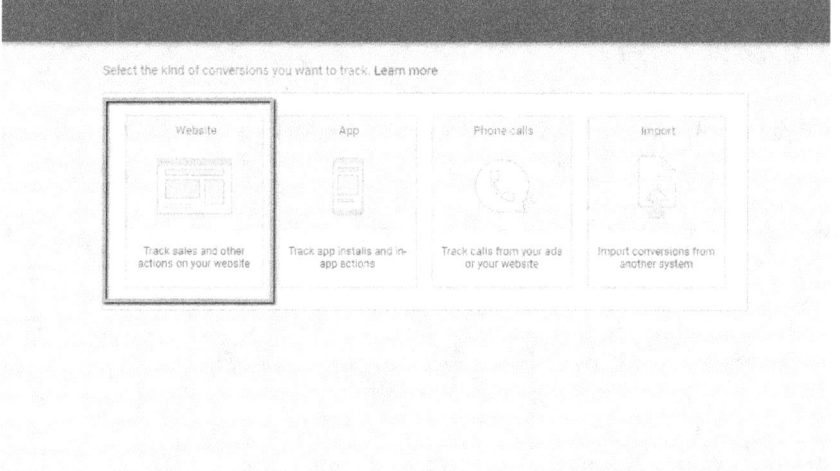

Then, set the parameters for the tracking you wish to engage in. The following example shows the tracking of conversions as they apply to Form Submissions. The tracking will go under the Lead category, it won't use a value, and will count a single lead per click for a span of 30-days.

Finally, apply the code to your form submission page and your tracking will go live.

How to Use Google's Keyword Planner

We reserved this section of the book to discuss Google's keyword research tool, which is the cornerstone of most SEO keyword strategies. Using this tool, you will be able to precision-target your digital campaigns for even greater results.

Imagine finding a keyword that was massively popular and yet had no competition. You'd be able to rank right away with a term like that! Those are the kinds of results the Keyword Planner offers.

Keep in mind that the planner's data could change as time goes on, as technologies become more advanced, and as Google alters its business approach.

Instead of focusing so much on how to use the platform, which we will of course provide instructions for, pay attention to the ideas behind the how-tos, so that you can roll with the punches and keep the research coming regardless of how much Google changes the game.

To access the keyword planner, visit your Google AdWords account and click on Tools, then Keyword Planner in the drop-down menu.

What the Keyword Planner Delivers

Keyword Research: Find out which of your keywords are viable for all your campaigns by viewing traffic data, competitor data, traffic estimators, and more.

Ad Groups: Find out which ad groups are best served to prospects and patients.

Bids and Budgets: Find out how to set your daily bids and establish budgets based on local trends and competitor data. Keep in mind that these will only be estimates, but they should serve as a guide to propel your AdWords campaign forward.

Match Type: There are three essential type of keyword searches. Broad match, which is characterized by the search term by itself; Exact Match, which is what you are looking for when you put the keyword in brackets; and Phrase Match, which is characterized by quotes on either side of the keyword.

Broad match is like searching for "dentist in Austin" and getting results for both dentist and Austin. This type gives you the most general search results. The search may also include synonyms and related words as Google attempts to understand what you are looking for.

You can also use broad match modifiers by using a plus sign in front of words (with no spaces in between, like +cosmetic or +implants) to enhance your search, and the results will yield all the pages that use those terms in any order.

Exact Match is like searching for "cosmetic dentist in Atlanta, GA" and getting results for only those sites that were crawled and found using that exact term in that exact order and with no other words being used.

Phrase Match is like searching for "cosmetic dentist in Austin that accepts Aetna insurance" and getting only those searches that use that exact phrase, or something very close to it.

The broader your search, the wider your marketing message will reach, but the less targeted it will be. Test the various match types to keep whittling your list down and find the most viable keywords that will give you the best results for your ad budget.

Searching for New Keywords

To search for ad groups and keywords from scratch, click on the tab Search for New Keyword and Ad Group Ideas within the Keyword Planner dashboard.

Here Google encourages you to describe your products and services.

Start with a phrase that not only describes your dental office, but that also separates you from all the other professionals vying for similar keywords. Remember to use geographic modifiers, such as, "Austin cosmetic dentistry" or "general dentistry in Beverly Hills."

Next, enter your practice's website URL and a category that is relevant to your practice. As with most Google products of this type, the moment you start typing your category, Google will try to predict what you are trying to say. Choose your categories based on the suggestions you are given, as those are usually the most searched within the AdWords system.

At the bottom of this initial form, you will notice a spot to indicate a number of filters you might use to narrow your keyword research down even further. You can select the country, language, and network to search for, as well as enter negative keywords.

Use the filters as you see fit, such as only searching for keywords that get more than 100 searches per month or only those keywords that offer at least 1,000 impressions. You can include words, exclude words, and basically customize your search however you see fit.

When you are satisfied with your criteria, hit the button Get Ideas and you will be taken to the Keyword Results page.

At the top of the Keyword Results page is a tab where you can select ad group and keyword ideas.

Ad group ideas will provide you with the most popular ad groups in your category, a list of the most popular keywords within those ad groups, and other vital information.

Average Monthly Searches: This number lets you know just how popular that ad group or keyword is. The higher the number, the more popular the term tends to be, and the more competition it is likely to have.

Competition: This represents the level of competition the ad group or keyword enjoys in three increments: low, medium, and high. The lower the competition level, the easier it will be for your practice to rank for the ad groups and keywords for which you plan to optimize.

Suggested Bid: No more guessing how much to bid and hoping that your ads show up for relevant searches. This number considers all the other advertisers bidding for that keyword and yields a monthly total that will give you a leg-up in the keyword bidding war, particularly if your competitors fail to use the Keyword Planner tool.

Ad Impression Share: This number considers your location and chosen ad network and predicts how many impressions and clicks that keyword is likely to share.

For those keywords that show a high percentage of impression share, you might want to click Add to Plan, which will place your favorite terms into a separate compartment, kind of like putting a product you like into an ecommerce shopping cart.

Monthly Searches: If you look closely, there is an icon that looks like a tiny graph directly in front of the search number. Hover over it and you will be able to view the average search volume for that ad group or keyword over the past few months. This helps you identify any trends in keyword searches. If one particular keyword shows an uphill swing, like Invisalign for instance, you'll certainly want to take advantage.

Add to Plan: Here you can implement, remove and edit new ad group ideas before you incorporate them into a planned or ongoing campaign.

When you have successfully put together a plan that you are sure will give your dental Internet marketing campaign a boost, click on the button Review Estimates.

Keyword Planner Estimates and Review Plan, New Ad Groups and Keywords

This section allows you to see the clicks, cost, and impressions per day that the ad group or keyword gets, as well as other details like the average position on the search results page and the overall cost to your AdWords budget.

You can search, test, and upload as an Excel or CSV file any ad groups or keywords that you wish to examine.

Existing Keyword Lists

Earlier you brainstormed and compiled a list of dental keywords, and you have been using those terms throughout your basic and advanced Internet marketing campaigns. This is the section of the Keyword Planner where you can copy and paste your list or upload it as a CSV file to check its viability.

Don't forget to list your keywords naked (Broad search), with quotes (Phrase search) or with brackets (Exact search) so that you can get the most accurate results.

When you are finished, click Get Volume to proceed to the results page.
To estimate the amount of traffic that you are likely to experience with your existing list of keywords, click on the link "Get traffic estimates for a list of keywords."

Again, enter your keywords naked, in brackets or quotes, or upload them as a CSV file and then hit Get Search Volume to continue.

Mixing and Matching for New Ideas

To combine and multiply your keywords, click on the menu item "Multiply keyword lists to get new keyword ideas." This allows you to combine your current keywords together.

Simply enter the first keyword you want combined, such as dentistry in Austin, with a secondary keyword that you want that keyword combined with, such as cosmetic dentistry in Texas.

When you are finished, click on Get Estimates or Get Search Volume to see the respective results.

We encourage you to use the Keyword Planner to get new keyword ideas and to narrow down your existing lists until you find those unique keyword terms that few other advertisers are pursuing.

Once you have a list of keywords that you know perform well, go back and start plugging those keywords into your on-site and off-site SEO campaigns.

Just make sure you maintain your keyword research so you can keep up with trends, buyer preferences, and current AdWords data.

How to Advertise on Facebook

AdWords is where your prime ad budget should be spent. After all, when your dental practice uses Google Ads, you're using keywords to target people who are actively searching for a dentist in your area.

For instance, Cynthia has cracked her tooth and is looking for a dental clinic in the Washington DC area that will accept an emergency appointment.

Cynthia, in pain and panicking, searches Google for "emergency dentist in Washington DC." Google instantly displays ads for dental practices that match her search.

Cynthia, in her dire need, just might end up clicking on one of those ads that promise instant dental pain relief.

That's Google's AdWords system. Facebook ads are different.

Facebook Ads are targeted to people's interests, not keywords. Think about how much data Facebook is able to collect on each user. Not only does it have names and birthdays, but it has phone numbers, interests, likes and dislikes, and demographics data that most advertisers would salivate over.

All of this information is readily available to Facebook every time a user logs in and interacts with the site, which happens to be the only way they can see Facebook ads.

The Facebook Ads platform continually collects and uses this information to target ads directly to specific groups of people. This is important when you're attempting to market to your ideal patient or Buyer Persona.

For instance, let's say that one of your dental prospects, Brian, gets engaged. Facebook knows about the engagement because Brian posted a "Life Event" on his personal page. Brian would be the ideal prospect to target with a Facebook ad displaying a special on teeth whitening or Invisalign. You can target people just like this using specific services in your Facebook Ads.

When it comes to Facebook advertising, mobile ads rule. In their 2015 Q4 Earnings report, Facebook revealed that 80% of their advertising revenue came from mobile. While this doesn't mean you should completely cut out desktop advertising, it does mean that your dental practice should seriously consider going "mobile first."

What Makes Facebook Ads So Effective?

Facebook ads offer dentists an excellent opportunity to appear in front of targeted prospects. The savviest dentists are just starting to utilize Facebook ads, but unfortunately, the majority are getting it wrong. Here is what you need to know to get the most out of this cutting-edge paid strategy.

Nearly everyone is on Facebook, which makes Facebook advertising one of the most efficient ways to place ads for your dental practice right in your neighbors' newsfeeds!

But not just any neighbors. By coupling user interests and location, Facebook can display your ads directly into the newsfeeds of users likely to need dental treatments near you.

A Facebook ad campaign allows you to explicitly target individuals in your location or neighboring area who may need a dentist. A pediatric dentist can target parents of young children while ads for oral cancer screening can be directed at older prospects in the same town.

You don't always need to be ultra-specific with your targeting. As long as you know the age and geographic area you wish to target, you can get excellent results.

How Do Facebook Ads Work?

One reason why Facebook advertising is so powerful is that your ads will accompany friend and family member posts in your audience's newsfeeds. This makes your ads appear more natural, causing people to click on them more readily.

While Facebook can help you attract loads of new leads, we recommend starting with a small initial budget. For best results, we advise you to start your Facebook ad campaign with $300 per month. As long as you track what works and what doesn't, your ad budget should be put to good use. You can always increase your budget as you become more skilled and in-tune with what your audience most wants.

Set up a Facebook Ad Account

Visit the Facebook home page (https://www.facebook.com/) and sign in using your Facebook account information you created earlier. Then, go to https://www.facebook.com/ads/manager. That's the dashboard where you will manage all of your Facebook ads.

Select "close" from the bottom left corner and take a few moments to configure your settings and billing information.

Next click on "Ads Manager" in the top left of your screen and then select "Settings." Update the information about your business, such as your account name, address, and time zone. You can also enable email notifications so that you receive regular updates regarding your Facebook ads status.

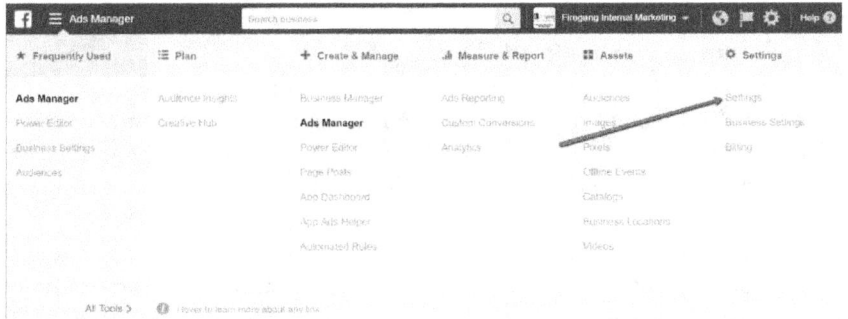

Now select "Payment Settings" from the left sidebar. Here is where you will fill out your billing preferences. We suggest adding both a primary and secondary means of payment. If your billing fails, all of your Facebook ads will be suspended, and you will have to go in manually and restart the ads once you have cleared your balance.

Facebook will bill you for your ads once you have reached a specific threshold. Typically, this starts at $25, then increases to $50, $100, and so on after your payments have cleared. You can set a limit to the total amount of money you want to spend on your ad account by editing "Control how much you spend."

Once you reach your spending limit, your ads will turn off, so you don't spend any more than the initial ad budget you set.

Double-check your account settings and billing options to ensure all of the information is correct. Then, you're ready to get started!

Creating Your First Facebook Ad

One of the most difficult aspects of Facebook advertising is knowing which groups to target. Here is where you are encouraged to revisit your Buyer Persona.

When searching for your ideal patient using Facebook's proprietary search engine, think about where the person might work, what interests he or she might possess, and what subjects might "entice the click."

Once you know, more or less, which Facebook users to target, you'll then want to consider which services you want to advertise. Instead of advertising just "dentistry," consider running ads for individual treatments, like teeth cleaning and dental implants.

How to Set up a Facebook Ad Campaign

Like AdWords, there are three different components to your Facebook ad. Each is important for organizing your ads, targeting different audiences, and measuring the results.

Campaign: This is the house for your Facebook ads. We recommend using a different campaign for each service you are advertising. For example, one campaign for dental implants and another for Invisalign.

Facebook Ad Set: Different ad sets allow you to target different audiences. If you're not sure which target demographic will resonate most with your ads, then a Facebook ad set will allow you to monitor and compare results. Your ad sets can contain a variety of ads types.

Facebook Ad: This is the actual ad that is housed within your ad set.

Now that you know the basic organization, you can continue to create your first Facebook ad.

Click "Create an Ad"

You'll find this button in the middle of your Facebook page. Note that you must be logged in to see this.

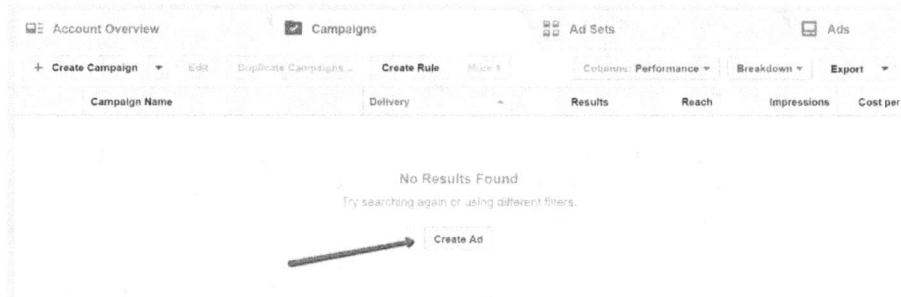

Choose the Objective of Your Campaign

Facebook offers you a variety of campaign objective types. There are actually ten in all. For now, you are going to choose "Traffic," which tells Facebook to send targeted people to your website.

For best results, limit your campaigns to a specific service. For example, if you want to advertise for implants and Invisalign, be sure to create two different campaigns.

After clicking on "traffic," you'll be prompted to pick a name. Name it "SERVICE - Traffic" according to what service is being advertised.

Pinpoint Your Target Audience

Now it is time to determine the audience for your paid Facebook ads. Here you will want to enter attributes that match your Buyer Persona, including the person's demographics information, likes, and dislikes.

You can target users based on their interests, Facebook groups they have joined, and Facebook pages they have liked. And, of course, you can filter users by their age, gender, and location.

Don't go too specific. It's best to go general and then narrow gradually than to alienate prospects right out of the gate. In fact, we recommend optimizing for area and age for now. Facebook is excellent at auto-optimizing, so let the platform do all the leg work for you.

How to Create A Custom Audience

You can also use your Facebook ad to specifically target those users who have already visited your dental website or signed up for your email list. This is a powerful way to nurture relationships with those people who have shown an interest in your services and offerings. This method is called retargeting, which can be highly-effective at spurring action in new prospects and current patients alike.

Selecting Placements

Now you have the option of selecting where your ads will display on Facebook. We recommend only selecting "Facebook News Feeds" and unchecking everything else as they are significantly less effective. Leave on "All Devices" so you show up on both mobile and desktop feeds.

How to Determine Your Ad Budget

Facebook allows you to select just how much money you would like to spend on specific ads.

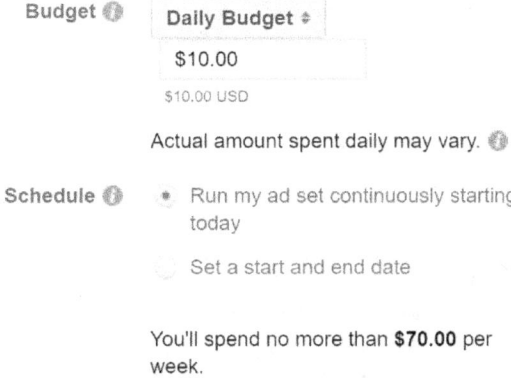

Theoretically, the more money you spend, the greater your reach and engagement. We suggest setting a daily budget to keep you from spending too much until your campaign is optimized.

Facebook will pace your spending to keep the ad running throughout the day. Start at $10 a day and then spend more once you measure what is working and what needs to be adjusted.

How to Create a Facebook Ad

Your Facebook ads should "speak" to your ideal patient, which is easier said than done. Using short and enticing copy and an image that captures the attention, your job is to entice people to click on your advertisement.

If you are new to ad copywriting, the tips below should help. Soon, you will be creating Facebook ads that convert just like an ad copy expert.

How to Write Enticing Facebook Ad Copy

You are allowed only a few words to get your point across when advertising on Facebook. The words you choose should be punchy, powerful, and relevant to your ideal patient's needs.

For best results, go for pain points. An ad about teeth whitening can ask simply, "Yellow teeth?" And an ad about tooth extractions can say, "Tooth Fairy Approved."

Your headline will garner the prospect's attention, then your ad must reel them in and hook them.

Use your imagination and try to come up with new and innovative ways to speak to your audience's problems, then present your ad as the relief they so desperately seek.

Here are a few other ad copy examples to attract a dental-centric Facebook crowd.

- Dental Implants: "Tired of Dentures? Get dental implants for only $X"
- Root Canals: "Painless Dentistry Done Right. The comfortable way to a healthier smile."
- Braces: "Beautify Your Smile....and improve your confidence with braces!"
- Invisalign: "More Confidence. Less Metal. Get a Free Invisalign Consultation!"
- Cleaning & Exam: "Got Bad Breath? Get a cleaning and exam for only $39!"

The Headline

Facebook allows 25 characters for the headline. Include a special offer, your service, and the name of your dental office, such as "Why Wait? Get Same-Day Crowns, only at **[Dental Office]**.

Ad Copy Formula

The proper text goes a long way. In fact, we have spent thousands of dollars perfecting the "ideal text" and finally developed a framework for how we structure long-text Facebook ads.

Paragraph 1: Explain what you are offering on an emotional basis.

Example: "Embarrassed about your smile? Invisalign can help."

Paragraph 2: Describe any long-term benefits of your services. For best results, include a statement of expertise.

Example: "Dr. Anderson can straighten your smile for improved confidence that lasts a lifetime!"

Paragraph 3: Tell prospects what they can expect by contacting you right this moment.

Example: "We just opened our calendars. Call today for a Free Consultation!"

The Image

The image you choose for your Facebook ad is extremely important. Dentists will often advertise their work with pictures of happy, smiling people. However, this image choice is usually unsuccessful. We've found that as much as 70% of a Facebook ad's success depends on selecting the right image.

When selecting photographs that depict people, take care to use images that depict where someone is right now, not where they hope to end up. The goal is for people to see your image and think "that's me." The highest converting photos are often pictures of the actual product.

Your imagery needs to be clean and professional. Don't clutter up the ad with arrows, offers, and text. Instead, get straight to the point, such as depicting a large picture of teeth to advertise dentures! Ads that are unique stand out, which is precisely what you want on Facebook.

Facebook offers a free image library you can use to design your ads, so always start there. You never know when you might find the ideal ad image to attract your audience.

Pixabay (https://pixabay.com/) and Pexels (https://www.pexels.com/) are two other sources that are excellent for finding Facebook worthy ad images.

Call-to-Action Button

Facebook offers a variety of Call-to-Action buttons such as Learn More, Contact Us, and Download. Select the button that most accurately applies to your offer. You can even try testing ads with no CTA buttons at all.

How to Track Your Facebook Ad Results

Once you have one or more Facebook ads up and running, you can optimize your ads by testing, testing, and then testing again.

Your Facebook Ads Manager will let you measure the success of your ads over time. At first, all the metrics can seem confusing. However, you can distill the information by only paying attention to the following figures.

Engagement: This is the metric that determines if people are liking, commenting on, and sharing your ads.

Performance: This metric describes the number of actions that have been taken by your audience as they pertain to your ad objective. For instance, if you designed your ads to entice patients to book an appointment, your Performance metric will let you know how many appointments were indeed booked as a result of your Facebook ad campaign.

Clicks: This metric represents the number of clicks the ad has received, as well as its click through rate (CTR) and cost per click (CPC).

Don't forget to test your ads often, including ad copy and your choice of images. For best results, don't be afraid to test different offers to determine which ones inspire more action.

Images: When selecting images for your ads, use real men, women, and children. Of course, your ad may not call for any people at all. Use your judgement and experiment to find images that may strike a nerve.

Audience: Your Buyer Persona may be off slightly, even after all your research. For that reason, you are encouraged to experiment with varying ages and other demographics to uncover any interested audience segments you may otherwise have missed.

The Anatomy of A Successful Facebook Ad

In our experience, there are five critical factors to every successful Facebook ad.

Business Info: Ensure that your business name is filled out and spelled exactly as it should to make it easy for new patients to find you.

Ad Text: This is the ad copy that will be displayed above your image. Keep it short, as you are only allowed 25 characters. There are tools that allow for more leeway, but it's better to be brief and get right to the point when advertising.

Image: This is the most important part of your ad, so invest in professional photos or use stock photos. Make sure your image is the proper size for the ad type and placement you are using. Otherwise, the image may appear cropped or skewed in users' newsfeeds.

Headline: Research shows that the most popular Facebook Ad headline length is only four or five words long. Don't write a book. Instead, explain why the prospect should select your ad for clicking, such as "Stop Tooth Pain" or "Get Braces for Less."

Call-To-Action: Facebook gives you a variety of Call To Action (CTAs) options, but we generally suggest you use "Learn More," which directs the person to your website.

Advanced PPC Marketing—the Possibilities

With your first AdWords campaign and Facebook Ads running, you should start receiving clicks to your website. Over time, and after enough data has flowed in, you will be able to identify certain advertising trends. Pay attention to these trends so that you can capitalize on them.

Like we mentioned before, you might begin to notice that most of your ad traffic is coming from tablet computers. Likewise, you may notice that most of your traffic happens between nine in the morning until 12 in the afternoon and only on weekdays.

As an AdWords and Facebook advertiser, you have many variables at your disposal that you can use to further hone your advertising skills and get more out of advertising budget.

You can, for instance, set your ads to run at certain times of the day and in certain areas. You can even rotate your ads and test them. You can run reports, set data filters, and tweak your ads until they are bringing in the traffic and leads you expect.

Keep in mind that we have only discussed Pay-Per-Click advertising, which is only one type of online ad. There are also display ads (among others). One type of display ad we feel is important to mention are retargeting ads.

The Power of Ad Retargeting

A common theme you will notice in this book is that proper marketing takes time. Whether you choose to hire a marketing company or go with the DIY approach, you shouldn't expect to receive an influx of new patients from the moment you publish your brand-new website to the web.

In fact, most studies show that prospects require seven or more interactions with your dental office before they are ready to commit. That's a lot of relationship building! How can you stay on patients' minds so that they always select your practice over the competition? One way is to "retarget" your audience with display ads.

What Are Retargeting Ads?

The primary difference between a regular online display ad and a retargeting ad lies in the target's past behavior. Retargeting ads are aimed at those individuals who have already visited your website. When that visit occurs, a bit of data is placed on the user's computer called a "cookie." That cookie allows your ads to follow your prospect across multiple platforms, from Facebook to Google to YouTube and elsewhere.

In other words, retargeting ads only display for those individuals who are most likely to be interested in your dental office, enhancing your chances of receiving a click.

Ad retargeting is critical for those high-value treatments like implants, where prospects may still be weighing their options. Your ads displaying at every turn for the prospect will keep your office top-of-mind when it finally comes time to schedule. That may take three, six or seven times, but eventually, your ad may get clicked.

How Do Retargeting Ads Work?

To set up a retargeting ad, you must put a unique pixel (or tracking code) on your website. This pixel remembers those people who have visited your dental website. (More specifically, it places a cookie in the user's web browser to remember them.)

When that occurs, any users who have already visited your website will then see your paid ads on other online platforms.

It is possible to set up retargeting ads for platforms such as Google, Twitter, Facebook, and YouTube. Each of these platforms has instructions for installing this pixel on your website.

What Do Retargeted Ads Look Like?

There are multiple ways to use retargeting ads to grow your dental practice. The two platforms we will focus on here are Google and Facebook.

Google refers to retargeting as "remarketing," but the overall premise is the same. These are the ads that you usually see at the top or bottom of your Google search results. They may also display as banner ads on other websites or embedded as text links. However, AdWords remarketing will not go into effect until you achieve 1,000 hits to your website within the same 30-day window.

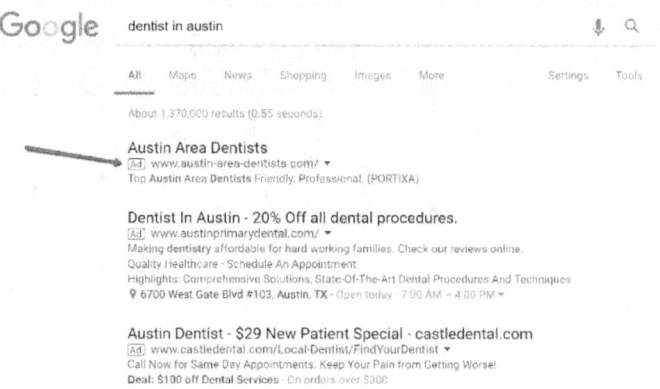

Facebook retargeting ads show up in users' news feeds or on the right-hand side of their Facebook pages. Few dental practices are taking advantage of retargeting ads, yet they can be a game-changer. Get ahead of the competition by using retargeting ads to start attracting your ideal patients today.

Learn how to create Facebook ads that get clicked. Download your Free Insider's Guide today!
http://www.firegang.com/book-bonuses/

Sample Facebook Newsfeed Ad

Many people suffer from dental anxiety preventing them from enjoying a great smile. Schedule a consultation with us to learn how we can make you comfortable during your visit.

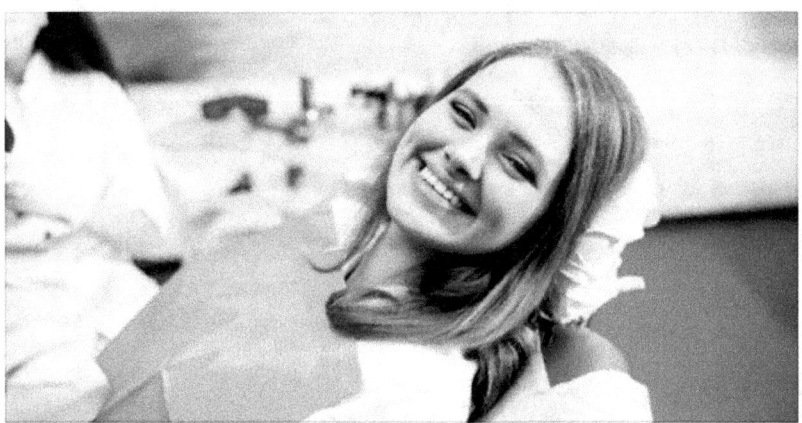

Sedation Dentistry - Your Visit Will Be Painless
Learn about the options ->

CHAPTER 14: PATIENT RETENTION & REENGAGEMENT

Attracting New Patients Vs. Retaining Patients

Much of this book has focused on attracting new dental patients to your office, for a good reason. Without a constant influx of new patients, your practice will not grow, and you won't achieve your major or SMART goals.

However, it is equally important to reengage with your current patients while retaining every patient on your roster. Every day, your competitors are trying to steal away your loyal patient base. This chapter is designed to keep your patients always coming back for more.

Do You Know The Lifetime Value Of Your Dental Patients?

Your patients are your most valuable asset. But it's not just the number of new patients your dental office attracts that matters—it's the total profit that those patients deliver over time that can make or break your business. In order to enact a successful dental marketing campaign (and calculate your return on investment), you need to know how valuable each patient is.

Learning Your Customer Lifetime Value (CLV)

Customer Lifetime Value is a prediction of the total worth of a client to a business over the entirety of their relationship. CLV is a crucial marketing measurement for any business, but especially for relationship-driven businesses like dentistry.

Think about your ideal patient. The person doesn't just schedule a routine check-up and then disappear. Instead, he may choose your dental office for all his dental needs throughout his lifetime, from cleaning and root canals to dentures and implants.

Your ideal patient depends on you to maintain his healthy smile for years on end—and all of those services can add up to some serious money.

What Is The Lifetime Value Of A Dental Patient?

No two dental practices are alike and, as a result, lifetime value will vary for each practice depending on the location, services offered and the effectiveness of the marketing strategy.

You often hear $10,000 thrown around as the magic number for the lifetime value of a dental patient. Derek Naylor, a dental practice consultant, claims a slightly more optimistic estimate at $22,000. At the top of the spectrum, True Dental Success believes that the CLV of a dental patient falls around $45,000 over a 20-year lifetime!

Given the variables between estimates, we suggest taking the time to calculate the CLV for your particular dental practice. Here are a few points to consider.

Lifelong Relationship: What is the total length of time (in years) that the average patient spends with you?

Average Annual Value: What is the revenue you make from each patient on an annual basis?

Client Referral Value: How many patients does the average client refer?

To calculate the lifetime value of your average dental patient, use this formula:

Average Annual Value x Lifelong Relationship + Client Referral Value = Lifetime Value

Let's break that down. First, determine how much the average patient spends per year. If most patients come in twice per year for cleanings and exams and spend $400 each time, then the Average Annual Value of your patient is $800.

Now we need to know the lifetime of your average dental patient. If you're not sure, use an industry average of ten years. We can plug that into the first part of our Lifetime Value Calculator and see that, so far, the patient's lifetime value is $8,000.

Average Annual Value ($800) x Lifelong Relationship (10 Years) = $8,000

But we're not done yet. Let's say the average client refers two new patients over their lifelong relationship with your practice. Each new patient is worth an additional $8,000. For two patients, our Client Referral Value is $16,000.

Go back to our calculator:

Average Annual Value ($800) x Lifelong Relationship (10 Years) + Client Referral Value ($16,000) = A Lifetime Value of $24,000

While you won't be able to predict the lifetime value of a dental patient down to the exact penny, as long as you know the average behavior of most of your patients, you should be able to get realistic data.

Still with me? Number crunching isn't always glamorous, but taking the time to monitor your new patients and get a prediction of their total lifetime value is critical to the success of your dental practice.

How to Maximize Your Patient Lifetime Value

Consistently Provide Quality Service: Never underestimate the value of over-delivering on your services and nurturing your relationship with your patients. Treat every patient like a VIP, and you can rest assured that your patients will keep coming back to you for all of their dental needs.

Acquire The Right Patients: To maximize the value that your patients are providing over time, you will want to ensure that you are acquiring the patients *you* want. These are the people who will say "yes" to complicated cases, and who have the insurance or income to pay for pricey procedures. Luckily, directing patients to these premium offerings is easier than you think.

Now that you know the real value of your dental patients, your practice can make more informed marketing decisions that will lead to your highest return on investment. And if you can increase the lifetime value of each patient, your dental office will experience steady profit gains, allowing you to finally achieve your long-term goals.

3 Keys to Improve Dental Patient Retention

Holding onto your current patients should take importance when implementing your marketing strategy. You can hold onto your patients, first and foremost, by treating every new patient like royalty.

One of our clients offers a complete 120-minute new patient exam which includes: a comprehensive exmaination, x-ray, and cleaning. The dentist has experienced such a massive positive impact from this tactic that he has vowed to never sacrifice this extensive new patient exam.

Setting this kind of precedence makes your patients feel at ease. They'll know they can put trust in your office and that they'll be well taken care of. Make it a priority to make your patients feel like a priority, and it'll differentiate you from your competitors.

Because the simple fact is, a new patient's first experience with your office should be unforgettable. Treat them with the red-carpet experience and your patients will surely come back when it's time.

Don't Stop There

Even if you treat your patients like kings and queens, they will still be eager to leave by the time the appointment is over. That's the nature of the game.

However, before each patient leaves, make sure you've scheduled a follow-up consultation. You might also want to implement a walkout statement. These tactics ensure that your patients leave feeling as though they have had a terrific experience.

A Follow-up Appointment

No patient should leave your office without being offered a follow-up appointment. These appointments help drive profits and improve retention rates while also keeping your patients healthy and happy.

Scheduling follow-up appointments can be tricky, particularly since patients are reluctant to schedule appointments more than a month away. On the other hand, arming your receptionist with the right words and a little persuasion can do wonders.

For example, your staff should always be using open-ended questions, such as, "You're due for another appointment in March. Dr. Anderson can see you on Wednesday the sixth or Friday the eighth. Which works better for you?" Avoiding yes or no questions makes it a lot harder for your patients to brush you off.

A Walkout Statement

The second item patients should get before leaving your office is a private walkout statement. These statements give the patient a quick summary of their dental health, records, and status, including their payment history, credit card payments, and insurance details.

The statement can also give a rundown of the treatment provided. By providing each patient with a general and honest overview of their information, they'll feel that your office is open and receptive to them, which encourages trust and ultimately leads to higher patient retention.

An Excellent Experience

This point cannot be emphasized enough. Your patients should always feel as though they have had an exceptional experience.

Unfortunately, a lot of people dislike or distrust their dentist. This doesn't mean your staff can't go out of their way to make patients feel more comfortable and less anxious along the way.

Be personable and ask specific questions so that patients feel comfortable throughout their entire visit. Ask them how their appointment went and ask questions, like, "Did your dentist see you on time?"

Oftentimes, patients simply want to discuss small issues or relieve their anxieties. Getting to voice their concerns to a caring staff member could be what defines their entire experience. Either way, listening to patient feedback and responding accordingly is a great way to enhance the patient experience and continually improve patient care.

Reconnecting with your patients after every appointment is fundamentally important for retaining them as loyal patients for life.

Focusing on Patient Retention and Re-engagement

There are other ways that you can focus on patient retention without wasting excess time and resources, such as practice management software.

Practice Management on Autopilot

Until A/I becomes more sophisticated, you will still need to partner with a marketing company like ours to see significant results. However, we often use software to make our jobs easier. We would like to tell you about a particular platform that could drastically improve your bottom line.

Sikka is a practice management system that syncs with your current system to display key business information in an actionable format.

The program allows us to send re-marketing campaigns to inactive patients that exist within your practice management database.

Furthermore, you have eight separate actions you can put in place to reactivate and invigorate inactive and active patients alike. Here are some other features this amazing platform offers.

- **Invite patients to bring their family members**
- **Reach out to patients who have outstanding treatment plans**
- **Notify patients of remaining insurance benefits**
- **Reach out to patients absent for longer than 7 months**
- **Reactivate inactive patients by offering an incentive**
- **Offer Invisalign (as a special)**
- **Offer Dental implants to patients wearing partials**

Any successful customer-based business prioritizes customer retention. Providing a great first-time experience is the first step across all industries. Getting software that remarkets or provides 6-12-month cleaning reminders is the next step.

Staff can then run customizable reports using this software to pinpoint no-shows and others who may be disengaged. These patients can then be discussed during meetings, and time can be set aside to call and email any patients who may require extra attention.

CHAPTER 15: TRACKING, TESTING & TROUBLESHOOTING YOUR CAMPAIGN

Tracking Results and Return-On-Investment (ROI)

By far the largest benefit to digital marketing is that you can track every touchpoint a visitor makes as they traverse the journey from lead to patient.

Just like the security system on your building can alert you if a person tries to access an entry point like a door or window, with *analytics tracking* you can see searchers who saw your online ads, who clicked on your ads, who clicked on your organic search results, who has landed on your website, and who has called you from the phone number displayed on your site.

While you cannot always identify the person by a face or name, you can determine the following details.

- ➢ The zip code and country the person resides in
- ➢ Type of device used
- ➢ The person's sex and gender, in some cases
- ➢ And what time of day the web visit occurred

Few other forms of marketing allow for such extensive tracking, and that makes digital marketing an invaluable form of advertising for dental professionals.

Without the ability to track results and successes, failures and attempts, and dollars spent and earned, digital marketing wouldn't be nearly as powerful.

FIREGANG FACT: Tracking, while important for digital marketing, is not a fix-all. Knowing how to track results and how to decipher the data is just as important as the act of tracking itself.

The reason we track our digital marketing campaigns is to discover what's working (and what's not). The first thing you should do when you want to measure the performance of a particular campaign is to identify one or more

Key Performance Indicators or KPIs.

Establish Your Key Performance Indicators

A KPI is any measurable element that determines the effectiveness of any aspect of a particular campaign. Put simply, it's a milestone reached, and a small goal won.

Here are a few examples of some KPIs you may wish to establish for your own campaigns.

> - **The amount of traffic that lands on a page**
> - **The number of people who were referred by social media**
> - **The number of leads that dialed the number on your site**
> - **The number of online forms that were submitted**

It helps to think of KPIs as "results" from click to call, though we shouldn't discount those patients who email or come on in.

To track your KPIs, we recommend Google Analytics.

Google Analytics

Google Analytics can get confusing fast. In the beginning, you are going to have all this data coming in, which will seem like nothing more than numbers and figures at first. Soon, however, you will begin to notice trends and patterns. It's then that you will be able to use those patterns over time to optimize and improve your results.

But let's be honest. More than likely, you will not be testing your campaigns all on your own. Your marketing agency will be in charge of that. Still, it is important that you know where to look and, most importantly, where to focus your efforts for maximum return on investment.

What About Return on Investment (ROI)?

Return on investment is the ultimate measure of your campaign's success. It's what you hope to get out of this whole thing, after all. Before you start crunching numbers, it helps to look at your campaign bit-by-bit.

Start by focusing on the various channels your campaign uses to attract phone calls, such as SEO and paid ads. Then gauge if the incoming phone calls to your office are being converted into appointments.

If there is a problem, we recommend that you troubleshoot your campaign by working backward. Check the phones, scheduling process, and then test website conversions. All of this will help you determine *how* your campaigns are performing and *what* you can improve.

Important KPIs to Track with Analytics

Your Analytics dashboard may seem a bit bare at first, but you will be provided with all sorts of data once your online marketing campaigns have received consistent attention. You can customize your dashboard any way you would like so that it displays any data you prefer, but the default data will work perfectly for now.

In one glance, you should be able to determine some or all of the following metrics.

Search Times: In a single glance, you can determine how many people are searching for you by month, week, day or hour. Being able to determine intense flow trends can help you concentrate your marketing efforts to coincide with those times.

For example, you may find that Saturdays and Sundays, which typically enjoy the most click-through rates, are really hot for Facebook referrals so you may choose to keep a staff member on-hand and active on Facebook during those times.

Site/Page Visits: Most marketers are initially interested in the overall number of visitors that land on their site. However, dig a bit deeper, and you will be able to determine how many people landed on your individual pages. Knowing which pages are most popular will allow you to see what works. You'll also be able to pay added attention to those pages that may be lagging.

External Referral Sources: This metric determines the status of your off-site SEO efforts by determining where most of your traffic originates, such as from other websites, social media profiles, directories, or plain old Google SERPs.

Production: Production refers to the amount of revenue earned from each patient. Whether they are new or returning, each patient's treatment cost equals your production amount. Additionally, other indicators fall under production and help designate where you should focus efforts including production per visit, new patient acquisition, and new patient visits.

Call conversion percentage: Call conversion percentage is the rate at which your dental staff can book appointments per inbound call.

Track Your Phone Calls

Google Analytics can't track your phone calls, but third-party systems can. We recommend coupling your call tracking data with your Google Analytics data to compound your efforts.

Call tracking tells you what portion of your calls are coming from organic SEO, paid ads, and social media. Along with the data your staff collects over the phone, in emails, and in person, you can gather invaluable data that can help to improve your conversion rates. For instance, if you've trained your staff to ask, "How did you hear about us?" then you are constantly compiling data that reflects where your efforts are working.

The Truth About Call Tracking Phone Numbers

Phone call trackers are automated programs that enable you to detect who is calling, what time they called, and exactly what was said. In some cases, you can have the conversation printed out into an easy-to-analyze text document.

Google Voice is a good example of a call tracker. You can use your own phone number, or you can get a Google Voice phone number. You can opt to receive a Google Voice number that includes your local area code, for example.

Call trackers like these are great, and they offer tons of data that can be analyzed to further improve your marketing efforts, but they can also hurt your local search rankings unless they are used properly.

Earlier we mentioned that local SERPs were largely supplied from the big three data aggregators, yellow pages sites, and other directories; you spent a lot of time ensuring that the information on those platforms was accurate and consistent.

Many of those platforms look to determine if the phone number you use is consistent with the address you list as your practice location. If the phone number and address don't line up, the platforms—and particularly Google—will think that you are trying to game the system. This could drop you down a few notches in the local SERPs, or it could take you off the first page altogether. Just a word of warning.

The correct way to use call trackers is to use a technique known as Dynamic Number Insertion. This is a call tracking method that displays a unique phone number on your website based on certain variables such as the keyword the visitor used to find you.

Dynamic Number Insertion is used by inserting a snippet of JavaScript into your website's code. Since your actual phone number is hard-coded into your website, your local SEO won't be affected. Yet visitors will see your call tracker phone number, allowing you to determine who called, when they called, and what was said.

Another option is to present your call tracking number on an image without alt-text. Since the image won't be crawled by search engines, your local SEO will remain the same, and you'll still be able to track your callers each time they call.

Whether you use call trackers or not, you should still train your staff to ask every caller how they heard of the practice and where they received the phone number. We also recommend recording phone calls to ensure that the proper phone policies are being followed.

Only by tracking phone calls can you accurately set and assess your KPIs as they relate to all telephone calls coming into your practice from your online marketing efforts.

Timber Dental is one client who benefited greatly from phone tracking and staff training. In fact, we were able to increase their call-answer rate to a whopping 95%! And, thanks to our marketing training team, we helped their staff capture a number of 5-star reviews to improve the office's online reputation.

By listening to calls, and having your team answer calls properly, your office can achieve similar results.

Run Regular Analytics Reports

We recommend that you run, retain, and study regular data reports—weekly, monthly, or every three months—to accurately assess where your digital marketing results are paying off the most. This will require the help of your staff members to gauge phone calls, emails, and visitors that walk through the door. Track everything, online and off, to determine what works and what doesn't. Then improve on what is working to bring even more well-paying patients into your office.

Track Patient Online Behavior

When the phone does ring, it is your goal that any staff member who answers the phone will be able to convert the caller into a brand-new patient. Whether the sale is closed or not, the results of the call or other interaction should always be recorded and analyzed so that the life of the patient can be tracked from the point of initial interest all the way to the act of paying for the first of many dental appointments.

In doing this, you can detect patterns forming. For instance, you may find that most of your patients are locating your website through Facebook and then calling your practice from your website. By understanding these associations, you can focus your energy and efforts to improve the number of leads that you receive and close.

Calculate Your Return on Investment (ROI)

Earlier, we calculated the lifetime value of each of your patients. Now that you know more about KPIs and analytics data, you will be in a much better position to calculate the amount of return your practice is earning on its marketing investment.

Let's assume that you spend $5,000 total on a domain name, hosting, and an AdWords account that features dozens of ads running in constant rotation.

To calculate your rate of return, you will take the number of new patients that you have earned from your campaign and multiply it by the LTV that you calculated earlier. Subtract that number from your online marketing investment and divide that number by your digital marketing investment.

Your formula may look like this:

(New Patients x LTV) − (Investment) ÷ Investment

For example, if you gain 12 new patients through your online marketing efforts, you earn an LTV of $1,400 per year per patient, and you spend $5,000 on your digital marketing efforts, your rate of return would be 236%.

We recommend you set up another tab in your online marketing spreadsheet to track your patient acquisition costs and rate of return, along with all of your other report data.

Test and Tweak to Improve Conversions

Rarely do Internet marketers get everything perfect right out of the gate, despite how much research they may have been conducted beforehand. This is why studying your analytics figures is so vital to your overall marketing success. If you know what to look for, your figures basically provide you with detailed instructions on how to make your campaigns even better.

A/B Testing

This is a technique used by Internet marketers to improve campaigns involving two similar elements that are tweaked slightly in the hopes of delivering measurable results. For example, imagine that you have an AdWords ad that is performing slightly well, but you do not see quite as much traffic as you would like.

To test the ad, create a duplicate ad that will run at the same time of day to the exact same audience, but possibly on alternating days. The difference is that the second ad will have a slightly different headline. By testing the two headlines with the same audience, you can determine which one is most effective at enticing the click.

You can then keep that headline and test the body of the ad, for example, then the landing page that you send your click-throughs to, and so on.

Testing takes time to collect the proper amount of data. Whatever you do, don't become impatient and stop your testing early to tweak another aspect of your ad, or another element. You must handle your testing like a scientist. Change one variable, keep everything else consistent, tabulate the results, and then start again until every element has been analyzed—and optimized.

After enough time has passed and enough testing has been conducted, you will find those elements that your audience truly responds to, and your results will speak for themselves.

Improving Conversions

After a while, you will become obsessed with converting your prospects and patients at every turn. You will begin to see trends, such as when the phone is most likely to ring. With enough attention, research, and getting to know your audience, the elements you need to change, and the avenues you need to pursue to improve your campaign will become clear as day.

But what if things don't quite work as you expect? When you need a little help with your campaigns, it is important to have a digital marketing troubleshooting guide.

If you have problems, one of these solutions is sure to get your campaign back on track.

Visit Google Search Console

Google Webmaster tools is now Google Search Console. This platform can give you data similar to Analytics, in that you can learn more about the keywords people use to find you.

The primary difference between the two platforms is that Google Search Console will help you define the keywords visitors might be using to find your site while Google Analytics will tell you what visitors are doing once they land.

Google Search Console can give you invaluable information to improve your search rankings and the appearance of your search listings.

PageSpeed Insights

PageSpeed Insights analyzes the content of your web page, then generates suggestions to improve your website's load time.

Google Tag Manager

Google has been improving Google Tag Manager, which is their platform for easy implementation of different types of tracking tags you may want to add to your site. Tag Manager makes it easier to set up conversion tracking, site measurement, and event tracking, and it allows for much more granular insights by giving you the ability to set up tracking of very specific things that users do while visiting your site.

As an example, we've started adding tags to the phone number anchor tags <a> on our sites that are tracking clicks from users on mobile devices, since those users are more apt to use click-to-call than users on desktops.

We've also set up specific event tracking for individual special offers on the home page so we can determine which offers are generating more interest from users.

Each special offer button has a tag implemented that when a user clicks one of those buttons, an event is sent to Google Analytics. That event will then be labeled with the name of that particular special offer as seen in the image. You can add AdWords conversion tracking tags using Tag Manager, as well.

Google Tag Manager is a tag management system that allows you to quickly and easily update tags and code snippets on your website or mobile app, such as those intended for traffic analysis and marketing optimization.

You can add and update Google AdWords and Analytics from the Tag Manager user interface instead of editing site code. This reduces errors and frees you from having to involve a developer when configuring tags.

Name ↑	Type	Firing Triggers	Last Edited
Ft. Lauderdale Adwords Conversion tag	AdWords Conversion Tracking	Thank You Page trigger	2 hours ago
GA - Event - 500 off Dental Implants Click	Universal Analytics	Special Offer Three Button Trigger	22 days ago
GA - Event - Free X-Ray and Second Opinion Click	Universal Analytics	Special Offer Two Button Trigger	22 days ago
GA - Event - New Patient Special Click	Universal Analytics	Special Offer One Button Trigger	22 days ago
GA - Form Submit Tag - Book an Appointment button	Universal Analytics	Book Appointment Button form trigger	22 days ago
Google Analytics	Universal Analytics	All Pages	2 months ago
Hallandale Adwords Conversion tag	AdWords Conversion Tracking	Thank You Page trigger	2 hours ago
Sidebar Form Tag	Universal Analytics	Sidebar Form trigger	22 days ago

Troubleshooting Your Campaigns

If your campaigns seem to be floundering, if web traffic isn't quite coming your way, or if your visitors seem to bounce more often than not, it is important to keep the following troubleshooting cheat sheet close by.

Here are the three most common reasons your Internet marketing campaigns aren't performing and how to fix them to keep the conversions coming.

Symptom #1: Low Website Traffic Levels

Possible Fixes

Search for your keywords in Google to determine where your site is ranking in the search results. Click on the other sites that are outranking you to determine what elements you can test and tweak to boost your rankings.

Ensure that you are targeting keyword phrases along with geographic location modifiers, particularly in your website title tags, headlines, and subheadlines.

Use a responsive design that is mobile-friendly so that mobile device users get the web experience they are intended to receive.

Run a MOZ Local report to determine if your citations are accurate and consistent.

Run a PPC campaign that focuses on your local market.

Check that all of the links that point to your site are working properly and contain hypertext (the words that make up the link) that is relevant to the page visitors will be landing on. For example, a link that reads "dental implants" should point only to a page that discusses dental implants.

Look at your site traffic in Google Analytics. Are there any long-term trends? Examine traffic by channel (Acquisition > All Traffic > Channels) What are your top channels? Which channels are increasing? Which ones are decreasing?

If you see that your Paid Search traffic is decreasing, it's time to give your campaigns more attention. If your Organic traffic isn't steadily growing, you need to make sure your citations consistency hasn't slipped, and that your on-page SEO elements such as title tags and meta descriptions are as relevant as possible.

Symptom #2: Not Getting Many Calls, Emails or Office Visits

Possible Fixes

Check the calls-to-action that are listed on your website and individual pages. Determine if they could be stronger or more targeted to the actions you are expecting visitors to take.

Fill out one of your own contact forms to see if you receive any errors and to ensure all of your messages are getting through.

Click on every one of your website pages to ensure that they are working. While you are at it, check all links pointing to your site as well as internal links to ensure that they are complete and that they are leading visitors to the intended landing pages.

We live in a mobile-first world. These days you can expect more than half of your site's traffic to come from people using mobile devices. Is your site fully responsive? Does it look good and function well on your iPhone? On your friend's Android?

Check your content to ensure that it is targeted and of the highest-quality. Make sure all of your visitors are able to find exactly what they are searching for when clicking on your site and individual pages.

Run analytics reports to see which of your pages, ads, and other marketing messages are converting and where you can possibly improve things.

You may try placing a section on your website that asks, "Why Choose Us?" along with several bullet points that describe your practice's primary benefits. In our experience, this can really help with website conversions.

Place your practice specials and discounts right on your homepage and above the fold so that visitors don't have to search to find it.

Make sure you have trusted logos right on your homepage. These don't have to be above the fold, but they should be present if you hope to gain extra credibility.

Overall, ensure your visitors have an easy and stress-free user experience. You may even get a few opinions from trusted patients to determine possible fixes that could help your conversions improve.

Symptom #3: Web Prospects Aren't Turning into Appointments

Possible Fixes

Ensure that staff is properly trained and that all staff members who answer the phones are following the agreed-upon phone protocol.

Record your office phone calls and listen for anything that may be hindering the conversion process.

Train staff members to check and respond to practice emails regularly and to always use calls-to-action that convince prospects to call, submit, or visit.

Follow a lead-nurturing schedule that has your staff members calling leads on a regular basis. If you need extra incentive to do so, consider the studies that show that nurtured leads make 47% larger purchases than non-nurtured leads. In dental circles, that means more premium treatments that further expand your bottom line.

Symptom #3: My Paid Ads Are Ineffective

If you are running an AdWords campaign and not getting calls, it is a good idea to check your average monthly searches and impression share. Your average searches reflect the average number of times people have searched for a specific keyword and its close variants.

Naturally, how often a paid ad appears in the Search Network will depend on budget, approval status, bids, quality score, targeting settings, and the competitive landscape. By adding a column for "Search Impression Share," you can better quantify these variables with a single metric which reports the percentage of ad impressions received out of the total number of impressions available.

This is useful in quickly identifying keywords, ad groups or campaigns that are not generating impressions (and clicks) as often as they could. To remain competitive, your dental practice should appear more than 65% (or 2/3) of the time for non-brand keywords and more than 80% (or 4/5) for brand keywords.

Trends

Once you get your search volume results, you can further analyze these statistics by selecting options within "Search volume trends." This information helps you understand the impact of your keyword on specific segments.

CONCLUSION - WHERE TO GO FROM HERE

A successful marketing plan takes time, money, and expertise. Most of all, it takes the sense to say, "I can't do this all by myself!"

Let's be logical, you are already busy running your practice and serving your patients. Do you really have the time or expertise to run your own marketing campaigns?

Of course not.

So why are so many dental professionals tempted to try?

For many dentists, money is the biggest issue, but it doesn't have to be. Spending your own time on marketing takes you away from the main focus of your practice. Your patients will suffer from lack of attention, and your business will lose much-needed profits.

Yes, digital marketing a dental practice costs money. In fact, as we've shown, you should be investing at least 7% of your monthly income into your digital marketing budget if you hope to compete in your market.

But don't think of digital marketing as another expense of running your business. Think of the return you will receive. The more you invest in digital marketing over the long-term, the more revenue you will earn for your practice.

The best way to think of it is like this: Your investment in digital marketing can continue to pay returns, all while freeing you up to work on developing your core business.

Moving Forward

The best advice we could give you moving forward is to *act*. On the other hand, telling someone to "take action" doesn't always work.

But we leave you with this: If you've ever struggled to create a positive change in your life, like losing weight, quitting smoking, or learning a musical instrument, then you know that <u>knowing what to do</u> and <u>doing it</u> are two entirely different things.

While lack of action can be due to laziness or distraction, more often it is due to fear of taking a chance. It's easier to keep doing what you've been doing than risk losing something you've built from the ground up. This fear of losing something we value, be it money, comfort, routine, or feeling of significance, is the main reason practices fail.

So why is doing the right thing so difficult sometimes? We know what to do? Why don't we just do it?

The reason for most of our clients' inaction is analysis paralysis. Most dentists have some concept of the things that must be done to achieve the future they want, but self-doubt holds them back.

They may constantly ask, "Do I know enough? Am I ready? Is this the right marketing company? What if their system doesn't work?"

This is why changing your mindset is so important. You can't waste time obsessing over the risk of failure. If you don't take *some* action, you're going to stagnate, and your dental practice will suffer. The trick to moving forward is to identify what you can control and prepare accordingly.

Aren't you ready to start making your major and SMART goals a reality? Take action today and hire Firegang Dental Marketing. The future of your dental practice just may depend on it.

APPENDIX

The following sections will help you learn more about Firegang's digital marketing processes and methodologies. You will find resources on how to create effective ads, how to convert patients, and much more.

In This Section

- **Do You Know the Lifetime Value of Your Dental Patients?**
- **The Perfect Dental Facebook Ad Strategy**
- **How to Turn Your Front Office Staff into a Gold Mine**
- **Firegang's Website Conversion Checklist**
- **How to Make Your Marketing Budget Finally Work**
- **Sustainable Growth: How a Group Dental Practice Stabilized Their Future**

DO YOU KNOW THE LIFETIME VALUE OF YOUR DENTAL PATIENTS?

Your patients are your most valuable asset. But it's not just the number of new patients your dental practice brings in that matters. It's the total profit that those patients deliver over time that can make or break your business. To start a successful dental marketing campaign, you need to know how much *value* each patient brings to the table.

Once you know the lifetime value of each of your dental patients, you will be better positioned to maximize your revenue and skyrocket your business, all while building meaningful relationships with your patients.

How to Determine Customer Lifetime Value

Customer Lifetime Value (CLV) is a prediction of the total worth of a client to a business over the entirety of their relationship. CLV is a crucial marketing measurement for any business, but especially for a relationship-driven business-like dentistry.

Think about your ideal patients. They don't just come in for one routine check-up and then disappear. Instead, these patients come to you for all their dental needs throughout their lifetimes. They depend on you to maintain their healthy smiles for years on end—and that can add up to some serious money.

Calculating the Lifetime Value of Your Dental Patients

No two dental practices are alike. As a result, the overall lifetime value will vary for each practice, depending on the location, services offered, and the effectiveness of their online marketing strategy.

Some practices use $10,000 as the magic number for the lifetime value of the average dental patient. Derek Naylor, a dental practice consultant, claims a slightly more optimistic estimate. At $22,000, Naylor is at the top of the spectrum. True Dental Success believes that the CLV of a dental patient falls around $45,000 over a 20-year lifetime!

Given the large expanse that exists between those estimates, we suggest taking the time to calculate the CLV for your specific dental practice.

To do so, consider the following.

> **Lifelong Relationship:** What is the total length of time (in years) that the average patient spends with you?
> **Average Annual Value:** How much do you earn from each patient on an annual basis?
> **Client Referral Value:** How many patients does the average client refer?

To calculate the lifetime value of your average dental patient, use the formula below.

(Average Annual Value x Lifelong Relationship) + Client Referral Value = Lifetime Value

Let's break that down.

First, determine how much the average patient spends with you per year. If most patients come in twice per year for a checkup and exam and spend $400 each time, then the Average Annual Value of your patient is $800.

If your dental practice just opened and you are unsure of how long each patient will stay with you, feel free to use the industry average of ten years. Now, plug that into the first part of our Lifetime Value Calculator, and you get a patient lifetime value of $8,000.

Here's the cheat sheet:

Average Annual Value ($800) x Lifelong Relationship (10 Years) = $8,000

But you're not done yet. What if your average patient refers two new patients over their lifelong relationship with you? Each new patient is worth an additional $8,000. For two patients, your Client Referral Value would be $16,000.

Average Annual Value ($800) x Lifelong Relationship (10 Years) + Client Referral Value ($16,000) = A Lifetime Value of $24,000

Of course, these are just estimates. You won't be able to predict the lifetime value of a dental patient down to the exact penny. However, as long as you know the average behavior of most of your patients, you will be able to get a realistic idea you can work with.

Number crunching isn't always glamorous but taking the time to monitor your new patients to get a prediction for their total lifetime value is critical to your success as a dental professional.

Why Does Customer Lifetime Value Matter?

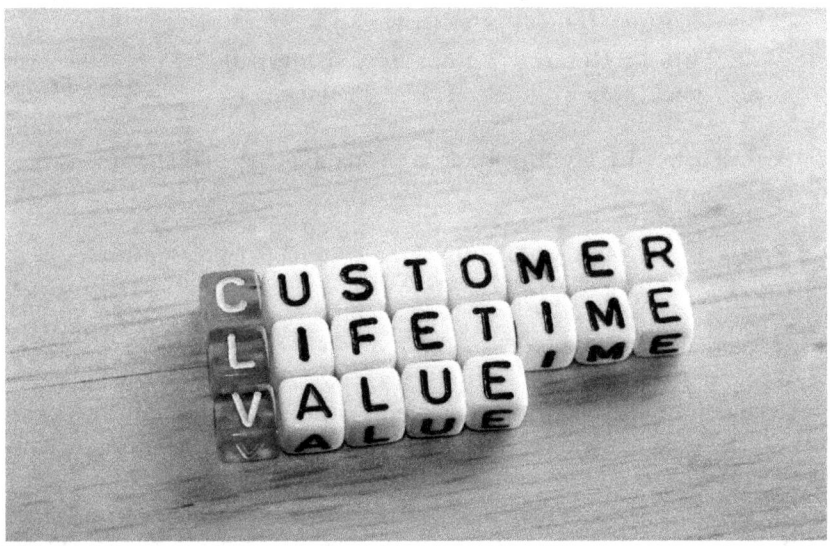

Once you know the lifetime value of a dental patient, you'll be able to make more informed marketing and advertising decisions. You never want to spend more money acquiring new patients than those patients will deliver to your practice over their lifetimes.

Knowing how much each new patient is worth to your practice right now will also give you a number to strive for. If you can manage to improve the lifetime value of your patients by a significant degree, your dental office will become more successful and valuable in case you ever decide to sell.

How to Maximize Your Dental Patients' Lifetime Value

Consistently Provide Quality Service

Never underestimate the value of over-delivering on your services and nurturing your relationships with your patients. Treat every patient like a VIP, and your patients will continue to return for all their dental needs.

Acquire the Right Patients

To maximize the value that your patients deliver over time, you will want to acquire the right patients. Those people who will say YES to complicated cases, and who have the insurance or income to pay for costly procedures. Luckily, directing new patients to these premium offerings is easier than you think.

Now that you know the real value of your dental patients, your practice can make more informed marketing decisions that will lead to your highest return on investment. And if you can increase the lifetime value of each patient, your dental office will experience steady profit gains, leading to a very successful dental practice.

THE PERFECT DENTAL FACEBOOK AD STRATEGY

4 Dental Facebook Ads for Attracting High-Value New Patients

Why Facebook?

Dentists are always trying to figure out innovative ways to reach new patients before the competition. The goal is to not only find new patients, but the best new patients that turn into high-value cases and loyal patients for life.

Marketing strategies that have worked in the past are failing to deliver new patients like they used to. This has left dentists searching for new strategies to reach out to patients in all new ways.

Due to the massive growth and success of Facebook Ads over the past few years, we wanted to find out if this tool could be utilized to attract the kinds of new patients that dentists need.

Five Major Questions Dentists Ask About Facebook Ads

- Are dental patients really on Facebook?
- Do Facebook Ads really work?
- Can Facebook attract high-quality new patients?
- Are Facebook Ads different than my Facebook page?
- What should I advertise on Facebook?

This guide is designed to answer those questions, provide you with our findings and best practices, and show you how to effectively run a Facebook Ad campaign.

Social Media Ad Revenue (Millions)

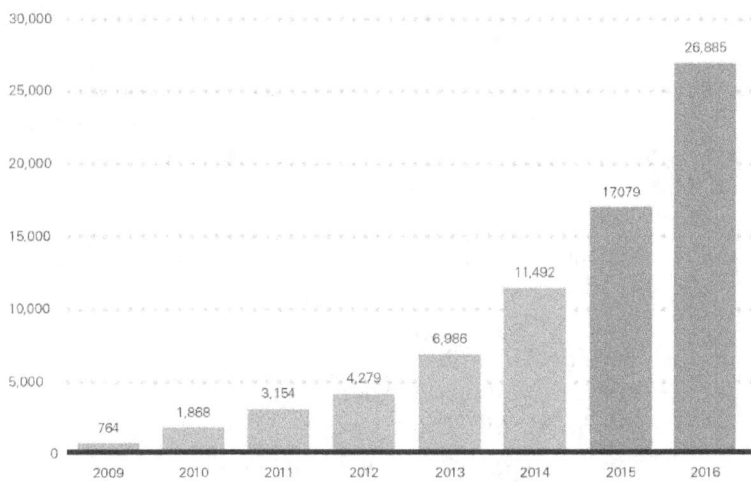

According to statista.com, businesses have been steadily increasing social media advertising spend. However, there was a huge jump from 2015 to 2016, with spending increasing to nearly $27 billion - a figure that's even more impressive, because just a few years ago that number was $0.

Why Facebook?

Facebook's Ads platform isn't new. It's been around since 2009 and continues to grow in popularity. According to The Guardian, more than 3 million businesses were advertising on Facebook as of 2016, actively turning Facebook users into customers, and the numbers have continued to explode ever since.

Still, one of the questions we frequently get from our clients is, "Are print ads in sources such as the Yellow Pages still relevant?" The data really speaks for itself.

From 2011-2013, 3.5 million people actively opted out of receiving the Yellow Pages and the publication's usage plummeted by 26%.

Yellow Page viewership continues to be in a sharp decline. To contrast, as of 2016, 88% of all local advertising was being delivered on mobile devices.

Not only that, but 1.5 billion mobile daily active users were on Facebook as of December 2016, an increase of 23% year-over-year. (Source: Facebook)

Facebook is growing while print ad platforms like the Yellow Pages are shrinking. Simply put, you want to display your ads where your patients are spending the majority of their time, which is – of course - online.

According to a report published by wearesocial.com, Facebook accounted for the lion's share of total social media user growth in 2016, increasing its footprint by over 363 million monthly active accounts, delivering year on year growth of 24%.

42% of small businesses report that Facebook is critical or important to their business growth (Source: State of Inbound Marketing).

- **363 Million Monthly Users**
- **3+ Million Businesses Advertising**
- **1.5 Billion Mobile Daily Users**
- **88% of All Advertising Now Delivered on Mobile**

Are Dental Patients Really on Facebook?

A little skepticism is understandable, especially if you haven't tried advertising your practice's services on Facebook before. Let us put your mind at ease: There are approximately 250,000 Facebook users within a 5-mile radius of most urban practices.

That means that, just by creating a few ads on the world's most popular social network, you can target a quarter million people in your immediate neighborhood RIGHT NOW.

Facebook allows you to segment your local market so you can advertise to your ideal patient, matching them with the services they're already looking for.

Even though Facebook Ads have been around since 2009, they are still a new strategy for most dental practices. The key is to use our best practices to set yourself up for success with every Facebook Ad campaign. That way you can be sure to attract the specific patients you want before your competitors realize they, too, can target 250,000 potential new patients in the same neighborhood.

Facebook Ads vs. Facebook Pages

A Facebook page and Facebook Ads are two separate entities. Your practice's Facebook page is a great way to connect with your existing patients, and can be a powerful tool for SEO, branding, and practice information. However, you don't need to be active on your Facebook page in order to run Facebook Ads.

In other words, Facebook Ad success doesn't depend on how often you post on your practice's Facebook page. In fact, you could literally NEVER post a single update to your page and still attract the patients you want on Facebook using the ad campaigns we outline in this guide.

Facebook Ads show up in newsfeeds. They DO NOT show up on your Facebook page. This means that the only people who will see your ads are people you choose to view them, and you don't need to worry about your Facebook page.

Facebook Ad

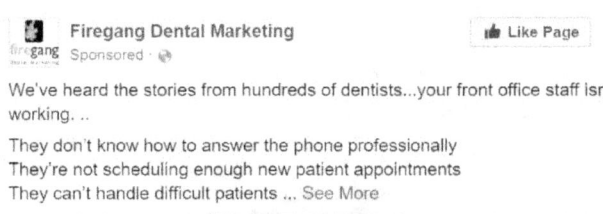

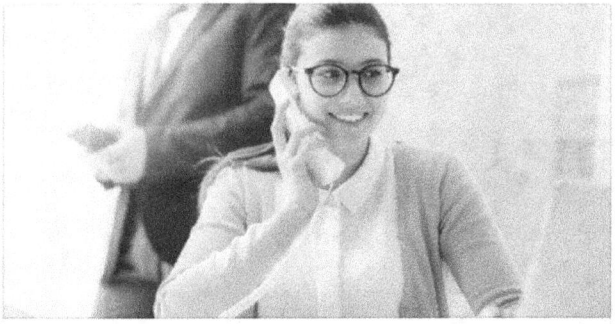

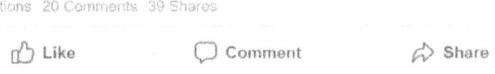

Facebook Newsfeed Post

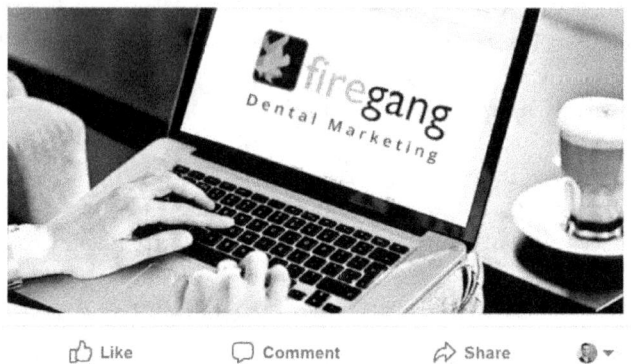

Facebook Ad Case Study 1: Invisalign

Target Audience: Women aged 25-55 within 5 to 10 miles.

What Worked

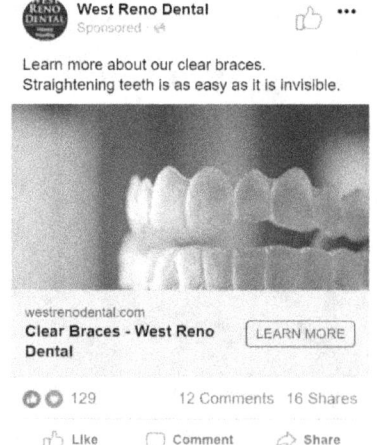

What Didn't Work

This is an example of an ad we tried that DID NOT work.

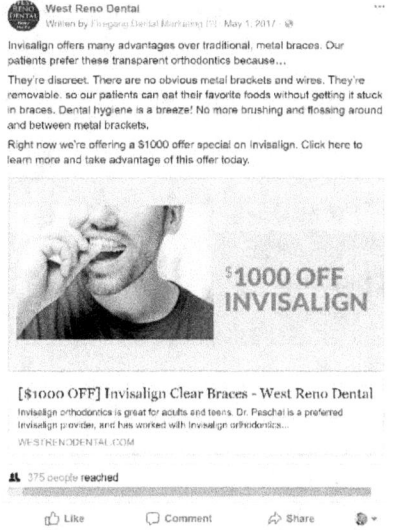

The Results

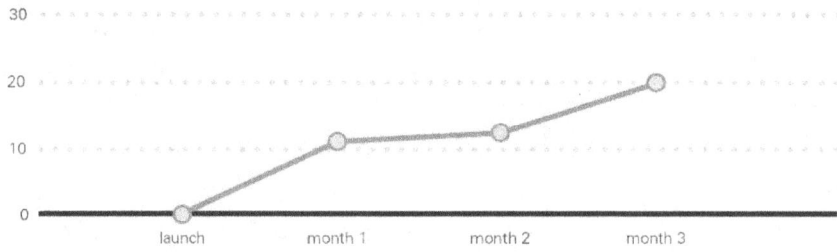

Ad Spend: $448
Timeframe: 3 months
Leads: 20
Cost Per Lead: $22

When we began running Invisalign ads on Facebook, we started putting ourselves in the mind of a potential patient, and we came up with many reasons why someone would be interested in Invisalign. Below are just a few of our findings.

We took the time to test each of these reasons through different ad styles, text, and images in over 20 different ads.

Through our testing, we were able to discover what Invisalign patients actually want. Because of that, we've been able to run the exact same ad for nearly 12 months, and it's still working to attract new patients for this client.

- ➢ They're removable
- ➢ They don't hinder oral hygiene
- ➢ They're comfortable
- ➢ They work (actually straighten teeth)
- ➢ It's an easy process
- ➢ They're customized for each patient
- ➢ They're discreet
- ➢ The treatment is invisible

The Top 3 Things Invisalign Patients Want to Gain from Treatment:

1) For the treatment to result in straight teeth
2) That Invisalign is a simple and easy process
3) That the treatment is invisible

Recommendations

If you look at our successful Invisalign ad on the previous page, you'll see that we combined these three elements into a single sentence. "Straightening teeth is as easy as it is invisible." One effective strategy on Facebook is to get your message across in as few words as possible.

How you present and talk about the treatment is also extremely important. When advertising Invisalign, we found that the word "invisible" is significantly stronger than "discrete" even though they imply almost the same thing.

Facebook Ad Case Study 2: Sedation Dentistry

Examples

Pro Targeting Tip: If your age range is too general, split your ads to target men & women.

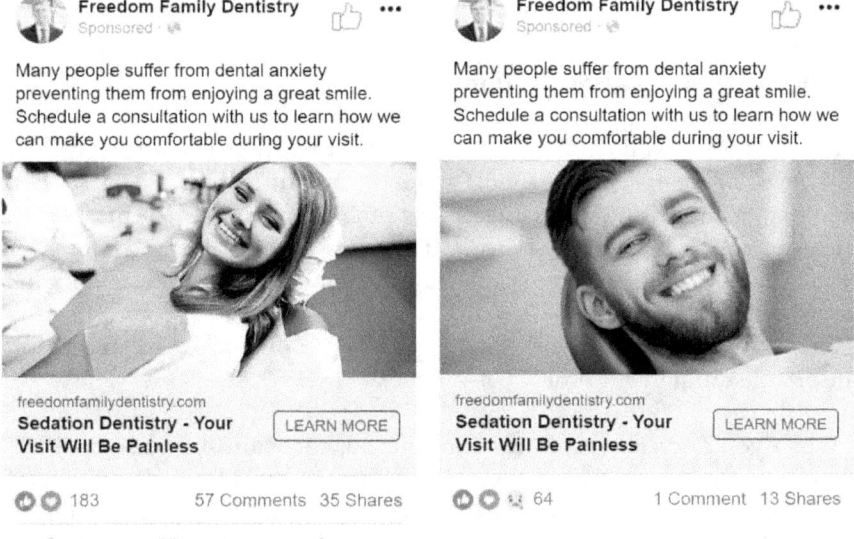

The Results

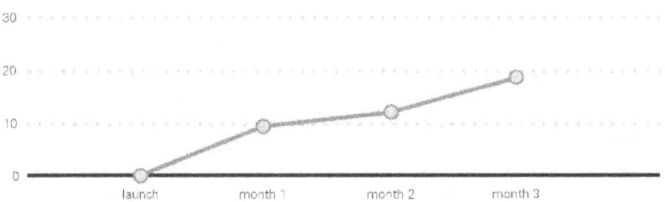

Spend: $599
Timeframe: 3 months
Leads: 19
Cost Per Lead: $31

Facebook Ad Case Study 2: Sedation Dentistry

Dental anxiety is one of the biggest reasons patients avoid coming to the dentist. Studies shared by Neuroscience Marketing and Colgate show that anywhere from 9% to 15% of Americans have a fear of the dentist. That's approximately 35 million people! By advertising sedation dentistry as a solution to ease that fear, you can reach patients who might have previously avoided your practice.

Emotional Advertising vs. Rational

Ad campaigns with emotional content performance twice as strong (31% vs. 16%) as ad campaigns with only rational content (source: Neuroscience Marketing) The reason our sedation ads work is because of their messaging. Instead of saying, "we have sedation dentistry... Check out the benefits of nitrous oxide," a purely rational message, the ads focus on the emotional response of a patient.

Our ads say, "Your visit will be painless" and "We can make you comfortable during your visit."

When you're creating the text for your ad, focus on the reasons WHY someone would want the service and less about the technical components of your offering. These emotional statements resonate with potential new patients much better than most rational or technical language.

Recommendations

Advertising sedation can be tricky because any age or gender group could find it beneficial. To be successful, you need to target your ads using a specific narrative.

The simplest narrative you can use is men vs. women. We created two sedation ads with identical messaging and targeted one ad toward women and the other towards men.

For the ad targeted toward women, we used an image of a woman, and vice-versa for the male-targeted ad. This small change massively boosted our conversion rates for this client.

Facebook Ad Case Study 3: Dental Implants

What Worked

Targeting: Men & women ages 35-64 within 3-5 miles of the practice.

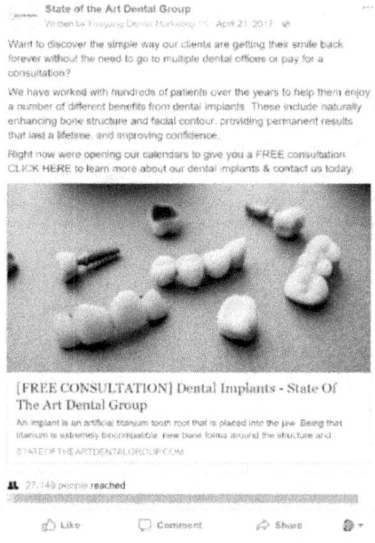

What Didn't Work

This is an example of an ad we tried that **DID NOT** work.

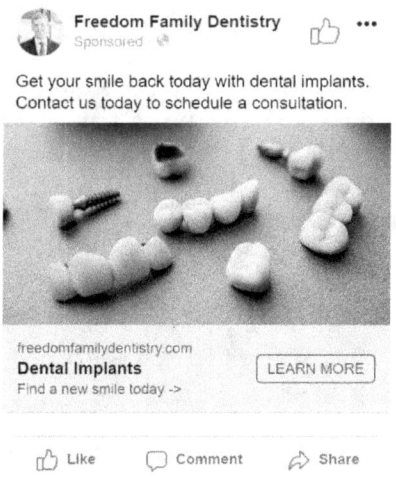

The Results

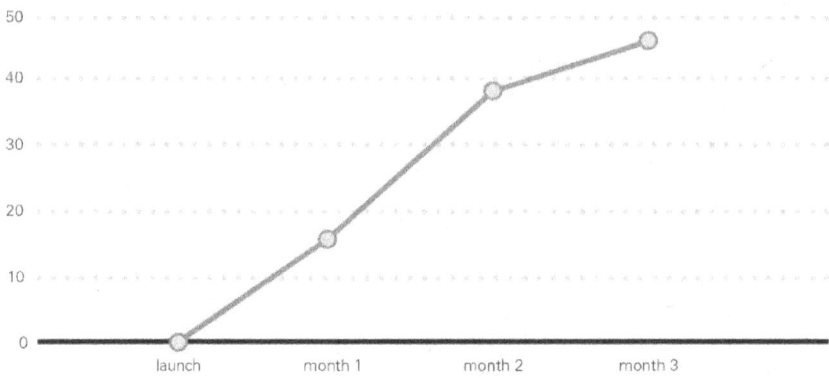

Spend: $1,035
Timeframe: 3 months
Leads: 46
Cost Per Lead: $30

We've had clients try to advertise dental implants with a short, simple ad basically saying, "Hey we have implants!" This absolutely can work on Facebook, but not always. Sometimes, in order to successfully advertise on Facebook, you need longer text to better explain the service you're advertising. Once we made this change with this dental practice's implant ads, their cost per lead went from $75 to $30.

Findings

The lesson is that the "right text" goes a long way. We spent thousands of dollars perfecting the "right text" and have developed a framework for how we structure long-text Facebook ads. Below is that exact framework:

Paragraph 1: Explain what someone can get emotionally.

Example: "Discover how our clients are getting their smile back."

Paragraph 2: Describe the long-term results a patient can experience from using your service. Also, include a statement of expertise.

Example: "...providing permanent results that last a lifetime while improving confidence."

Example: "We've worked with hundreds of patients..."

Paragraph 3: Tell prospects what they can get if they were to contact you right now.

Example: "We're opening our calendars to give you a FREE consultation."

Headline: Include a special offer, your service, and the name of your dental practice.

Recommendations

There are certain things you can and can't say in your Facebook ads. The most notable being that you can't say the word "you" in relation to something negative. The best way to get around this is to share anecdotal evidence from your own experiences. For example, "Discover the way our clients are getting a great smile."

For a full explanation, be sure to read our blog post, Writing Facebook Approved Ad Copy.

https://www.firegang.com/facebook-approved-copy/

Facebook Ad Case Study 4: Dentures

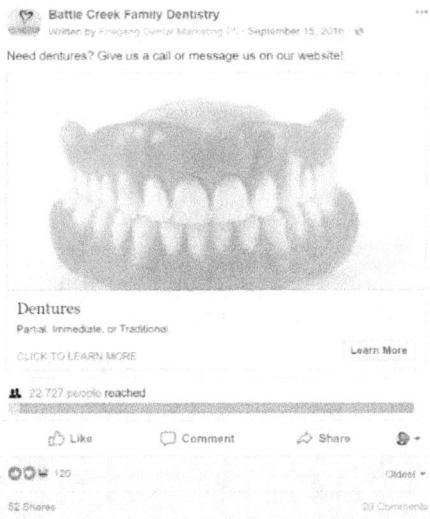

The Results

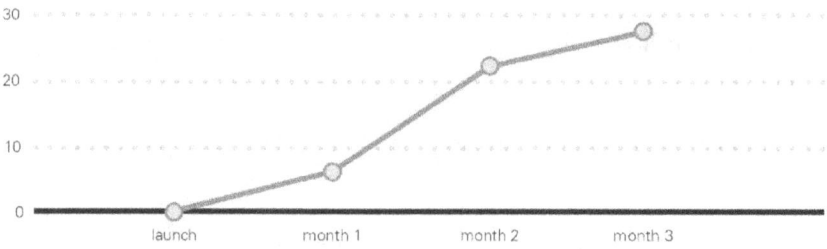

Spend: 449
Timeframe: 3 months
Leads: 28
Cost Per Lead: $16

Most of the success from this denture ad came from the image. The copy is extremely simple, but people know exactly what we're advertising because of the image. We split tested several different picture options, and this was the best because it's simple, clean, and doesn't look too gross.

Findings

The image you choose for your ad is extremely important. Dentists will often advertise their work with pictures of happy, smiling people. However, this image choice is usually unsuccessful. We've found that as much as 70% of a Facebook Ad's success depends on choosing the right image. Should you choose to show people in your ads, you need to use images which depict where someone is right now, not where they hope to end up. The goal is for people to see your image and think "that's me!"

Recommendations

The best converting images are often pictures of the actual product. Three of the four ads in this guide use pictures of the actual product, and that's why they're so successful. Your imagery needs to be clean and professional. Don't clutter up the ad with arrows and offers. When advertising dental services, you want to keep your images free of text.

Additionally, a big picture of teeth like the one we show in the Dentures ad example will stand out! It's so different that it's eye-catching, and this makes a huge difference.

Bonus Tip: Facebook Engagement

One of the bonuses dental practices get from running Facebook Ad campaigns is that they typically experience a grouping of organic, genuine comments. Potential and current patients often comment on ads and the key is for your practice to respond to these comments. As you can see below, people will leave reviews for you on your Facebook ads. You can't get this kind of natural engagement and social proof anywhere else. Social engagement like this can improve your reputation even better than a 5-star review on Google. It's the next level of "word of mouth," which is the social proof dentists need.

Facebook Engagement

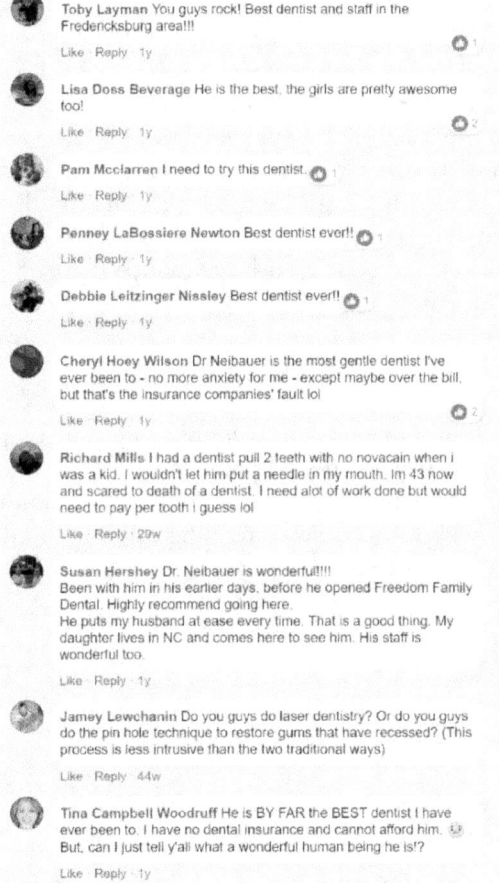

How to Find the Right Image for Your Ad

Finding the right image for your ad is extremely important. Facebook itself has a huge FREE image library you can use, so definitely start there when looking for the best image for your ad campaign. All of the images we used in the Facebook Ad campaigns included in this guide are available for free through Facebook's image library.

A few other sites that have fantastic free images you can use include:

- https://www.pexels.com/
- https://pixabay.com/

Top 3 Secrets for Attracting New Patients with Facebook Ads

Trust Facebook to optimize the targeting for your ad. Once you set up your basic target demographic, don't adjust them every day. It takes 3-5 days for Facebook to really optimize your ad, so give them time to make them work for you. Always target 5-7 miles around your practice. Having a dentist nearby is important to potential patients and they're going to be the ones most likely to schedule an appointment. Don't try to get patients to call your practice using a Facebook Ad. These ads work best when they're driving potential patients to your website. Let your website convince them to give you a call and book an appointment.

Conclusion

This is the end of this section, but only the beginning of your journey toward using Facebook Ads to attract the dental patients you want. With a clear plan to follow and solid execution, the way we've outlined in this guide, you should be able to focus Facebook's endless targeting options to attract the lifelong dental patients your practice needs to thrive.

HOW TO TURN YOUR FRONT OFFICE STAFF INTO A GOLD MINE

The strategies one dental practice used to increase new patient bookings over the phone by 61%.

Isn't it ironic that no formal qualifications, specific training, or certifications are required for a dental practice's front office staff? For roles that will make or break your practice, the front office staff members are often overlooked. How much of a gold mine is your front office staff?

What You'll Find in This Guide

- Best practices for hiring your ideal front office staff
- The 7 Golden Rules of phone answering
- What to say to create rapport with patients on the phone
- How to turn price shoppers into booked appointments
- Expert insights, phone scripts, and action plans you can use to avoid painfully common mistakes.

One of the practices we work with who has seen a drastic improvement in their new patient numbers is a multi-location practice based in Portland, OR. Before instituting phone training for their staff, they converted 46% of calls to appointments. After working to use these strategies consistently they began converting 75% of their calls to new patients in just 3 months.

New Patients - Three Month Growth

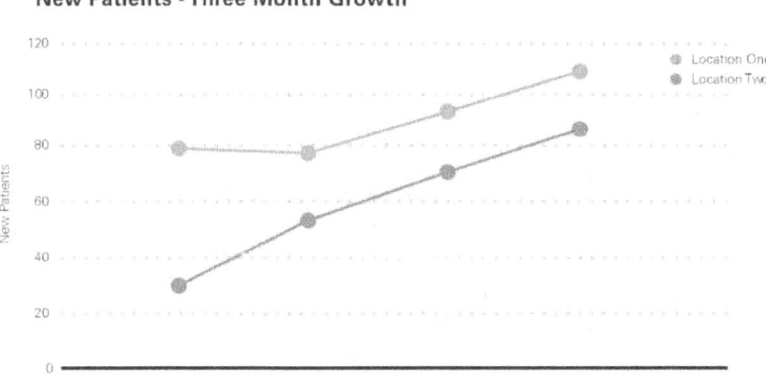

Step 1: Research

The first step in creating a strategy to hire and train a more effective front office staff is to research your competition. Go online and Google dental practices in your area. Put together a short list of the most successful practices, then grab a notepad and pen and take notes while you call each office. Pay attention to the demeanor of the person who answers the phone, what words they use when greeting, whether they tried booking an appointment with you and what incentives they offer to encourage potential new patients to come into the office.

Before implementing your own strategies, it's a great idea to seek inspiration from your competition. Combining any ideas relevant to your practice with those found in this guide can take things to the next level.

We want to give you some examples of how to set yourself up for success hiring future front office staff members.

Every time you find yourself in the hiring position, let it be known that you expect a process of continual improvement on the following skills:

- **Advanced phone training**
- **Asking patients to leave online reviews**
- **Patient empathy and relationship-building techniques**
- **How to contribute to the practice's social media presence**
- **Occasionally learning new software and/or phone systems**

A basic understanding of dental procedures, treatments and the time it takes to complete them Dental insurance plans (if your office takes them) and fees for treatment.

If you can set the expectation that professional development and continual learning are parts of the job, it'll be much easier to get your new employee on board. The best part is that setting professional development and trainings as being expected and required gets employees agreeing to engage in these activities from the start without it feeling like any "extra" work is being asked of them.

Step 3: Create Strategies

No one likes to feel unprepared for a job they must do and answering the phone is the primary responsibility of your front office staff members. With that in mind, put standard rules in place and provide your staff with scripts. Make sure you set aside time for employees to roleplay as patients, so they can be confident in their new phone skills. This will also give them a chance to ask any questions they have and help you head off common on-phone mistakes before they even happen.

The 7 Golden Rules of Phone-Answering

1. Always answer the phone with a smile, as it comes across in your tone of voice on the phone call.
2. Always ask for the caller's name at the beginning of the call.
3. Ask if you can put someone on hold before doing so.
4. Always answer within 4 rings as an absolute max or the person will already be thinking about calling the next practice.
5. Avoid a monotone voice at all costs, as it will bore people and lose their attention.
6. Never eat or chew gum when on the phone.
7. Never type, read or send text messages while on a call. Giving a patient your undivided attention is essential, especially when speaking to a potential new patient!

Sample Phone Script #1: The Basics

Let's start with something simple: everyone who calls into your office should be greeted with a basic, pleasant welcome:

Staff Member: "Good Morning, this is Susan at Happy Smiles Dental Clinic. How can I help you today?"

Quick Tip: As soon as the patient identifies themselves by name, the front office staff member should always address them by that name. This helps to build a personal relationship and shows respect. Make sure that if they transfer the call to another staff member, that they have the name and an understanding of why the person is calling.

Staff Member: "It was a pleasure talking with you today, Mr. Jones. Before I say goodbye, is there anything else I can help you with today?"

Make sure your front office staff understands that there is no exception to the rule of answering the phones in a pleasant and courteous manner.

Quick Tip: Even if you're dealing with an angry or frustrated patient, make sure your staff knows to keep their cool. Most angry patients will calm down if their concerns are listened to with respect and addressed quickly. If the staff member can't calm an angry patient, make sure they know they can come to you, a manager, or fellow co-worker for support in handling those difficult patients.

Sample Phone Script #2: Booking an Appointment

Staff Member: Good morning. Dr. Smith's Family Dentistry. This is Tracy. How can I help you today?

Patient: I need to come in for a checkup and get my teeth cleaned.

Staff Member: Great! Can I get your name and phone number in case we're disconnected during the call?

Patient: Gives name and phone number

Staff Member: Thank you. Ms. Jones, do you mind if I ask when was the last time you were in to see us?

This helps determine if this is a new or former patient without offending a former patient by not remembering them!

Patient: I think my last appointment was about a year ago.

Staff Member: After locating patient's record and confirming it is the right person by DOB or phone number. Have there been any changes to your phone or address since you've been last seen?

Patient: No.

Staff Member: Ok great, are you having any problems with your teeth or experiencing any pain we should know about when we do your cleaning?

Patient: I chipped a molar and it isn't causing me pain but has a jagged edge.

Staff Member: I'm sorry to hear that, but glad it isn't causing you pain. I can schedule an appointment for you to see Dr. Smith tomorrow at 3pm, will that work for you? Proceed to schedule the visit and always end the call thanking them for scheduling.

Sample Phone Script #3: Scheduling New Patient Appointments

Staff Member: Thank you for calling Dr. Lane's office. This is Joan. How may I help you today?

Patient: I just moved to the area and I need to find a dentist.

Staff Member: That's great! We're always excited to have new patients join us. I just need a little information from you before we schedule your appointment, is that ok? Get patient name, DOB, dental insurance (if they have it), etc.

Staff Member: [Patient Name], are you experiencing any pain or having any problems with your teeth?

Patient: No. I just need a cleaning.

Staff Member: Okay, great! Since you'll be visiting us for the first time, let me tell you what you can expect from Dr. Lane and all of us here in the office. Include whether they see the hygienist first, the dentist, what paperwork to bring with them, etc.

Staff Member: [Patient Name], Dr. **[Name]** has an opening in his/her schedule for an appointment on Thursday afternoon or Friday morning. Which would you prefer?

Patient: Thursday afternoon would be fine.

Staff Member: Perfect! I'll schedule you for Thursday at 2:00 p.m. Our office will also give you a call the day before just as a reminder. Before I go, do you have any other questions I can answer for you?

Sample Phone Script #4: The Follow-Up Call

Dental practices often miss out on retaining patients because they don't follow up post-appointment, especially when the patient was told they need to schedule a second appointment to receive another treatment (i.e. root canal therapy, a crown, etc.)

Set aside time for the front office staff each week to call the prior week's patient list (when appropriate) and make sure your patients don't slip through the cracks!

When calling, it is always best to speak to the patient directly. If your staff does need to leave a voicemail, have them keep it short, friendly and encourage the patient to call the office.

Staff Member: "Hi, this is Brenda from Dr. Hill's office. I'm calling to schedule a follow-up appointment from your **[date]** visit for your **[type of treatment]**. Do you have any questions about the treatment or cost for this visit?

If "No"

Great! Then, I have an appointment time available for you on _____ at _____, how does that work for you?

If "Yes"

Answer their questions and again, offer a date/time to schedule.

Quick Tip: If your staff calls a patient three times on three different days/times and still ends up with a voicemail, then send a letter or email to follow up instead.

Make sure the front office staff logs all calls, emails, and letters sent and results in the patient's clinical notes. This way if one of the doctors wants to reach out personally to a patient they can do so easily.

Three More "Golden Rules"

Try to avoid discussing prices over the phone. This is truly the most golden rule of any sales-based business. Patients will decline your service before they really know what you have to offer and why it's priced the way it is. Instead, try to help the patient understand that the best way to get an accurate price is by scheduling a consultation. If the patient still presses for a price, give them a price range. Even if the range is a large one ($300 - $800 for example), many times the patient will accept that information and schedule an appointment.

Never end a call without trying to book an appointment. Often, potential new patients are just a simple invitation away from visiting you and if your front office staff doesn't actively try to book appointments on every phone call, you won't secure half as many new patients. When offering to book an appointment, make sure to offer 2 different appointment times so the patient can easily choose which works for them!

Provide an Offer or Incentive of Some Kind

Consider offering a free checkup, a reduction in cost of teeth cleaning, free whitening with every new patient appointment, or other simple incentives to encourage patients to go ahead and book an appointment.

Warning Signs: Employee Behavior

Managing front office staff can seem daunting, but having a friendly, competent staff on hand to interact with patients is vital to your dental practice's success and growth. Keep an eye out for any of these warning signs in your front office staff members and make sure to address them before they become a problem.

Remember, never address a behavior issue in front of other staff. Instead, always set aside time to meet with a staff member one-on-one to address the problem and find a solution.

Attitude Check

Take a moment or two to observe your front office staff and see how they behave with your patients or potential patients. Are they happy, a pleasure to speak with, cheerful and bubbly? Or, perhaps they're cold; seem stressed, tired or just lack that customer care attitude. If you're seeing the latter, it's time for a conversation with your staff member, especially if this behavior seems out of character for them.

Body Language

See if your front office staff member is slouched behind the desk, perhaps with their arms folded in a defensive manner or using postures such as having a chin resting on one palm at the desk. Consider having a conversation if you feel their body language isn't welcoming to new patients.

Remember, you don't get a second chance to make a first impression. That statement might be a bit cliché, but it still rings true! For most patients the first impression they have of your practice is your front office staff.

Can you afford for them to have a negative experience?

By using the tips, scripts and strategies we've outlined in this guide, you'll be well set up to train your existing staff members to convert more calls into new appointments as well as set up standards for future hires.

If patients feel comfortable and well-cared for while in your office interacting with your front office staff, you'll convert more to lifetime patients who continue to give you referrals for years to come.

Firegang partners with dental practices in the United States and Canada using a variety of marketing initiatives to help generate new patient leads, including:

- Conversion-driven & mobile-friendly website
- Reputation management
- Online reviews
- Pay-per click advertising
- Organic search engine optimization

If you're ready to take the next step to grow your practice using a customized dental marketing strategy that works, schedule a complimentary call with our team, we'd be happy to chat with you.

FIREGANG'S WEBSITE CONVERSION CHECKLIST

Use the checklist and tools listed below to make sure your practice's website is designed to convert visitors to new patients.

Patient-Focused Information

- Short Sentences
- Concise Paragraphs
- List of Accepted Insurances
- 3rd-Party Lending Options
- Easy to Find Contact Info

Differentiators

- Financing Options
- Comprehensive Treatment
- In-House Services
- State-of-the-Art technology
- Free Consultations

Consistency

- Offers Listed on Homepage
- Contact Info on Every Page
- Address on Google Maps
- Hours Listed Correctly

Trust Factors

- Memberships & Associations
- Show Awards
- Include Staff Photos & Bios
- Google & Yelp Reviews

Give a Reason to Schedule

- Raving Testimonials
- Schedule "Buttons"
- Showcase Special Offers

Social Media Logos & Links

- Facebook
- Twitter
- LinkedIn

Special Offers

- Show on the Homepage
- List of Discounts/Specials
- Offers Expire Soon!

Is your website missing any of these vital pieces? If you're ready to take the next step to grow your practice using customized dental marketing strategy that works, schedule a complimentary call with our team, we'd be happy to chat with you.

Test Your Website's Display on All Devices

According to moboom.com, "Mobile First Web Design" is an approach that designs for smaller screens first, then adds more features and content for bigger and bigger screens.

This type of design is crucial for your website, since every year more and more traffic is coming from phones, tablets and smaller screens rather than desktop computers.

If your site is displaying well on mobile devices, it will translate as a better design to any larger device, too.

However, keep in mind that it's not just about screen size. The mobile-first approach means that the content on your site needs to be brief and to the point.

No rambling paragraphs of text or you'll lose potential patients very quickly.

Use the tips listed below to make sure your practice's website is designed the way it should be for mobile use.

Does Your Website Have Mobile First Design Features?

To find out, test your site with one or both of these online tools.

- http://mobiletest.me
- http://quirktools.com/screenfly/

Is It Easy to Contact Your Practice on Any Device?

- **"Click to Call" Phone Numbers on Every Page**
- **Click to Email Direct Link**
- **Is It Easy to Navigate on Mobile Devices?**
- **Mobile Menu**
- **Links Easy to Click Using A Finger**

- **Does It Load Quickly?**
- **Test with this online tool:**
  https://developers.google.com/speed/pagespeed/insights/

HOW TO MAKE YOUR MARKETING BUDGET FINALLY WORK

In this section, you will learn how to leverage your finances, time, and resources using online marketing to increase the number of new patients you attract each month.

According to The Bureau of Labor Statistics, 20% of small businesses fail in their first year, and 50% of small businesses fail in their fifth year. Unfortunately, this means many privately owned dental practices won't be around in 5 years, which means:

- **Fewer retirement options for dentists and staff**
- **Dentists having to work longer hours just to survive**
- **Smaller profits and even smaller paychecks**

This is why investing in marketing is vital to your dental practice's growth and success. Based on our 10+ years working with dentists in different markets across the US and Canada, we know that executing a consistent marketing plan is key to your dental practice's success.

If you aren't investing correctly in a strategic marketing budget, your practice could easily become a failing statistic. We understand that talking about budgets can be uncomfortable and awkward, but we'd rather have the tough conversation then set you up for failure and frustration!

In this guide we're going to give you:

- Industry suggestions for the proper marketing budget
- Formulas and tools for calculating return on investment
- Simple changes you can make to your practice to make it more attractive to new patients and easier to market

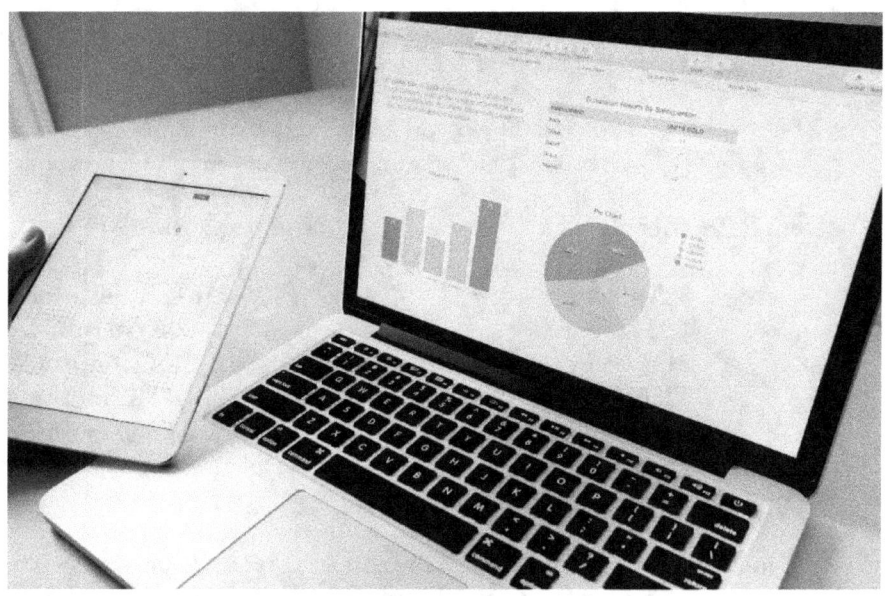

Where to Begin with Your Budget

Your marketing budget should be consistent with your business growth goals. If you want to aggressively grow your practice, that will require a higher digital marketing media budget. If you want to test the waters, aren't sure what the competition in your market looks like, a slow-growth path might be the best choice.

So where do you start? According to the Small Business Administration, businesses with revenues less than $5 million should allocate 7-8% of their revenues to marketing. Furthermore, the budget should be split between brand development costs (website, blog, sales collateral, etc.) and the costs of promoting your business (campaigns, advertising, events, etc.)

Entrepreneur Magazine recommends spending 12-20% of your revenue on marketing if you're a new company (est. 1-5 years) and 6-12% if you're an established business (5+ years).

According to DentalTown, many practices recommend at least 5% with some pushing 6-8% if they're in a competitive area. Firegang clients generally allocate a minimum of 5-7% of their revenue to spend on marketing in order to stay competitive. If our clients want to dominate their market and see rapid growth, we recommend they spend 10% of their revenue on marketing.

Still, there is no "one size fits all" when it comes to setting a marketing budget for your practice. Each dental practice is unique and there are many factors to consider when setting up your budget.

Below is a chart that can help you get started analyzing how much your practice should be spending on marketing based on your annual revenue.

Dental Practice Size	Recommended Budget
➤ $2M/year+	➤ $8.5K-$11.5K/month
➤ 1.5M/year	➤ $6K-$9K/month
➤ $1M/year	➤ $4K-6K/month
➤ $750K/year	➤ $3.5K-$5K/month
➤ $500K/year	➤ $2K-$2.5K/month

It's Not Just About the Numbers

Planning financially should be a big part of your marketing budget, but it isn't the only factor to consider. Your marketing budget should include 2 factors: finances AND marketability factors. Marketability factors play a huge role in attracting new patients and should be considered when creating your budget.

Remember that as a practice becomes more marketable and patient-centric, the easier it is to attract new patients. Here are a few things you can do to get your practice on the road to optimal marketability.

Marketability Factors

Consider staying open until 7pm instead of closing at 5pm. Or offer weekend appointments. According to a survey run by DentistryIQ, extended office hours during the week are important to 57% of those surveyed. And, nearly half of the patients surveyed look for dentists offering weekend hours!

Invest in tracking your calls. What good does it do to spend money to attract a new patient if your staff fails to schedule them for an appointment when they do call?

Invest in creating a website that isn't just "pretty." Of course, you want a website that is aesthetically pleasing, but remember: pretty websites don't necessarily convert visitors to new patients! Work with your marketing company to design a website created to turn visitors into new patient phone calls and appointments. This can be costly, but your website is the center of every marketing effort you make, so remember it is likely worth the expense!

Magic Smiles: Phoenix, AZ

Within 6-8 months of working with us, he was able to get the floundering practice he took over back on its feet.

The practice has grown, added a fourth location and this year, Magic Smiles, is projecting their fourth straight year of 10% growth.

"I know the initial price tag for marketing can seem high but remember on average for every dollar I spend on marketing, I get at least $10-$15 back!" – Mr. Daniel Morissey, CEO, Magic Smiles

Marketing Tools: Calculate Your Return on Investment (ROI)

Return on Investment (ROI) is a measure of the profit earned from each investment. Like the "return" (or profit) that you earn on your portfolio or bank account, it's calculated as a percentage.

In simple terms, the ROI formula is:

(Return – Investment) Investment

It is typically represented as a percentage, so just multiply your total by 100.

ROI calculations for marketing campaigns can be complex because you will have many variables on both the profit and the investment sides.

However, understanding this formula is essential if you want to produce the best possible results with your marketing investments.

Marketing Tools: Calculate Your Customer Lifetime Value

You can also use the Customer Lifetime Value (CLV) equation as a measurement to determine your ROI.

CLV is a measure of the profit generated by a single customer or set of customers over their lifetime with your dental practice.

You can determine your patient's average lifetime value by using this calculation:

Average Annual Value x Lifelong Relationship = CLV

(Customer Lifetime Value – Marketing Investment) Marketing Investment

For Example: Let's say your patient's average annual value is $800 and the lifelong relationship is about 10 years. That gives 1 patient a lifetime value of $8,000.

Use Your Marketing Budget to Guarantee Your Practice's Growth

If a dental practice eventually wants to get to $1M in revenue, creating a marketing budget is essential.

If you use the Customer Lifetime Value calculation, you can determine exactly what you need to do to get there.

Example: Assume that 1 new patient has a $1,500 lifetime value and if you want to bring in $1M annually, that means you need to see approximately 667 new patients in one year. To break that down even further, divide by 12 and you get 55 new patients per month. That's your target.

Dental practices often think that they're "saving" money by not spending money on marketing, but that's completely incorrect.

Think about it this way: by not spending that $300 per month on online ads you miss out on attracting 2 new patients per week, which means you're costing your practice $12,000 per month in revenue based on the assumed lifetime value of a patient.

Your practice just can't grow the way you want it to, the way you need it to in order to stay competitive, without making a calculated investment in marketing.

Review your marketing options with a strategic approach focused on helping your practice reach its overall growth goals.

Even if your marketing budget might be smaller than the competition, that does not mean you can't scale and grow with the resources you have!

Final Thoughts

Just spending money and hiring a marketing company isn't enough, you need to be an active part of creating a patient-centric practice that supports your marketing efforts.

As tempting as it can be when creating a marketing budget, remember that spending less doesn't actually save your practice anything.

Keep in mind that there is a cost for a lack of new patients each month…you're likely losing them to your competitors down the street.

You can try to cut corners and save money today, but in the long run, you will be better off in investing an appropriate amount to a marketing budget that actually works for your practice year after year!

Firegang partners with dental practices in the United States and Canada using a variety of marketing initiatives to help generate new patient leads, including:

- **Conversion-driven & mobile-friendly website**
- **Reputation management**
- **Online reviews**
- **Pay-Per-Click advertising**
- **Organic search engine optimization**

If you're ready to take the next step to grow your practice using a customized dental marketing strategy that works, schedule a complimentary call with our team, we'd be happy to chat with you.

Get a dental marketing strategy that helps your dental practice scale like never before. Visit us today at http://www.firegang.com/ **or call (800) 398-0979 for a free consultation.**

SUSTAINABLE GROWTH: HOW A GROUP DENTAL PRACTICE STABILIZED THEIR FUTURE

Discover how a multi-location dental practice increased new patients per month by 30% across 5 locations in less than 2 years.

Smile Design Dental is a group dental practice located in Florida. They became a client with Firegang in June of 2015. At the time, they brought on just one of their five locations (located in Coral Springs, FL) to see what results they could get from online marketing.

The practice's #1 struggle when they partnered with Firegang was their scattered online presence. They had five locations, with 5 names, 5 websites, and 5 individual teams marketing and managing each location.

The practice began to realize this wasn't working. Their branding and message was inconsistent. Patients couldn't find the right practice online since there were five different websites. Overall the focus of the dental practice was scattered.

Realizing they needed to unite their five locations under the Smile Design Dental brand, they brought their other four locations into the partnership with Firegang in April of 2016. That became the turning point for the practice.

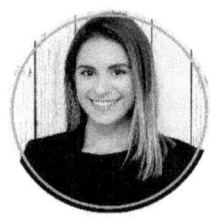

"It just didn't make sense to run 5 dental offices that belonged to the same group but had completely different names. I created a marketing game plan for our CEOs and it just made sense to make the big move and rebrand. It was the best decision we have made!— Daniela Velasquez, Chief of Operations — Smile Design Dental

By working with Firegang to create a unified marketing strategy and single focus, each of their locations have been able to see consistent new patient growth from every marketing channel they use.

In this case study, we will show exactly how Smile Design Dental continues to grow by using a consistent brand message and innovative dental marketing strategies through their partnership with Firegang.

Results

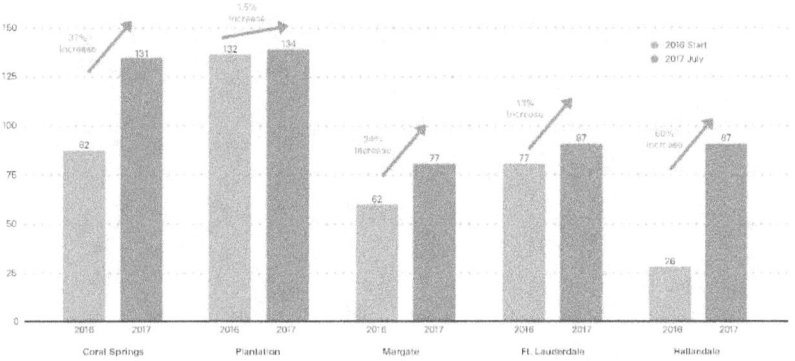

Over the course of 15 months (April 2016 – July 2017), Smile Design Dental had experienced an increase in new patients at each location.

Their Coral Springs and Margate locations both saw more than a 23% increase while their Hallandale location experienced incredible growth at a 60% increase.

Smile Design Dental continues to see sustainable growth at each of their five locations due to:

> ➢ **Unifying their locations under one consistent Smile Design Dental brand.**
> ➢ **Pipelining their scattered website traffic from five different websites into one patient-friendly website.**
> ➢ **Fixing their local citations for each practice's location.**
> ➢ **Continuing to ask their best patients to leave online reviews.**

Results

Steady Increase in New Patients Over Time

By pipelining Smile Design Dental's website traffic from five scattered websites (one for each location) into a single website, patients were able to find the practice easily, and organic website traffic surged.

Smile Design Dental still lists organic website traffic as the #1 reason new patients book an appointment with their practice.

Definition: Organic Website Traffic

This term refers to your website visitors who have found your practice's website as a result of unpaid search results. Visitors who are considered organic find your website after using a search engine like Google, so they are not "referred" by any other ad or website.

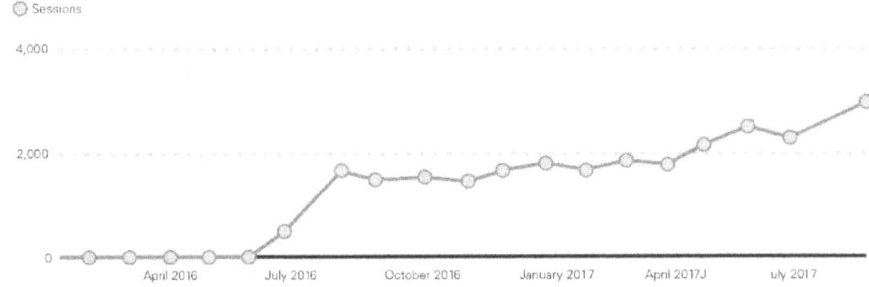

The business saw steady increases in organic website traffic beginning in July 2016, only three months after all five practices were brought on board with Firegang.

The site experienced an 81% increase of organic website traffic in 13 months. 315 (July 2016) to 1,735 (August 2017)

Smile Design Dental saw a 142% increase in users visiting the website over 12 months with a 216% increase in new visitors to the website over a 12-month timeframe.

Pipeline Website Traffic

The #1 reason Smile Design Dental has seen such continued, sustainable new patient growth across all five locations is because they unified all those locations onto one website.

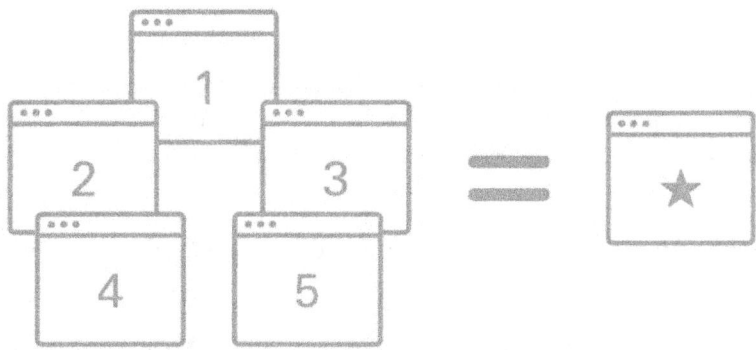

Unifying the practice's locations into one website dramatically improved their SEO rankings with Google, which led to an increase in organic traffic. SEO (Search Engine Optimization) is done in order to keep a dental practice's website competitive. Search engines like Google group similar types of websites (i.e. dental practices) together and compare them to each other to create a ranking. The higher a site's ranking, the easier it is for consumers to find.

In Smile Design Dental's case, their brand was spread across five different websites.

Each one of those websites was struggling to get to the top of Google's search results and were actually competing against one another for rankings.

Once the five websites were combined into one, it helped Google give it a better ranking and increase website traffic overall because every patient searching for Smile Design Dental went to one site.

Citations Improved the "Right" Way

Another vital step group dental practices need to take to ensure their SEO rankings aren't damaged in the transition is correcting and maintaining online local citations.

What is a Local Citation?

A local citation is any online mentions of the name, address, and phone number for a local business. Local citations can occur on local business directories, on websites and apps, and on social platforms.

Local citations help Internet users to discover local businesses and can also impact local search engine rankings.

To get the best local SEO results, multi-location dental practices need to have each location listed independently across multiple online business directories, as well as clearly state they are all unified under one brand.

Firegang treated each of Smile Design Dental's locations as an independent entity and start cleaning up and building at least 100 citations around each location.

"Cleaning up citations" means removing all online incorrect listings of past business names and past dentists associated with each of those locations. Each location now has its own local phone number and address clearly listed.

Smile Design Dental also added locations to their main practice name, which continues to be a huge factor in getting positive SEO rankings. For example, their Fort Lauderdale location officially became "Smile Design Dental of Fort Lauderdale." This is the same formula for all of their other five locations.

Smile Design Dental also has a Facebook page for each location as well as Twitter accounts. The practice doesn't need to constantly post to these accounts, but they do work to add additional credibility to local citations and improve the practice's overall SEO rankings. There are hundreds of websites that could list your dental practice as a local business, so it's important to make sure each of your locations are listed correctly, otherwise it can damage your SEO rankings.

5 Locations = 1 Website

Below you'll find an example of Smile Design Dental's unified website. The site was designed to make it easy for new patients to find whichever location is convenient for them and book an appointment while maintaining the consistent Smile Design Dental brand.

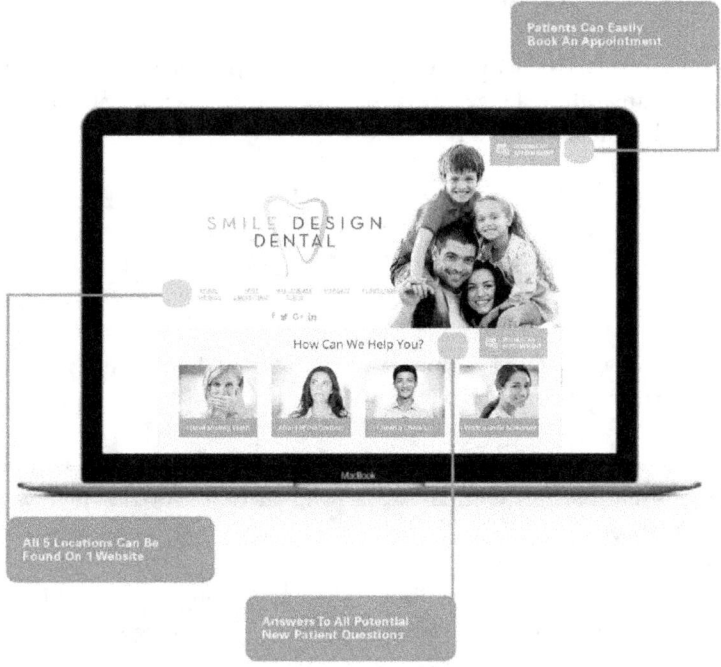

Recommendations

One Brand - One Team

Smile Design Dental is using a variety of marketing methods to attract (and keep!) new patients. However, their continued success can be traced back to that one crucial change they made back in April 2016:

By unifying their locations under one "Smile Design Dental" brand on a single website, each of their locations is clearly unified under one Smile Design Dental "umbrella." The logos are the same, the branding message is clear, and patients can easily find what they need because of this.

The second vital decision they made was to not only unify their locations, but also to bring every location in to be managed by a single marketing company. By doing this, Firegang was able to partner with Smile Design Dental and create a consistent brand message designed to attract new patients. This eliminated confusion for the practice as well as potential new patients.

Improved Online Reputation

Nearly 9 out of 10 people will call a dental practice with 5-star Google reviews over any other. This means that new patients are mostly interested in a doctor with a stellar online reputation.

A strong, positive online presence is vital to growing your dental practice, and online reviews are a large part of that. Positive online reviews equal trust for new patients and are social proof that you provide a high quality of dental care.

Make sure you're giving them the attention they deserve and making them an integral part of your practice's marketing plan.

Firegang worked with each location to drive Google reviews up. As of July 2017, Smile Design Dental had a total of 886 Google Reviews across their five locations.

Each location has a 4.6 or above star rating on Google with the Fort Lauderdale location set as a 5-star rating with 190+ reviews.

Compared to nearby dentists, Smile Design Dental of Ft. Lauderdale exceeds the competition in online reviews. This makes them appear as the #1 chosen practice in the area.

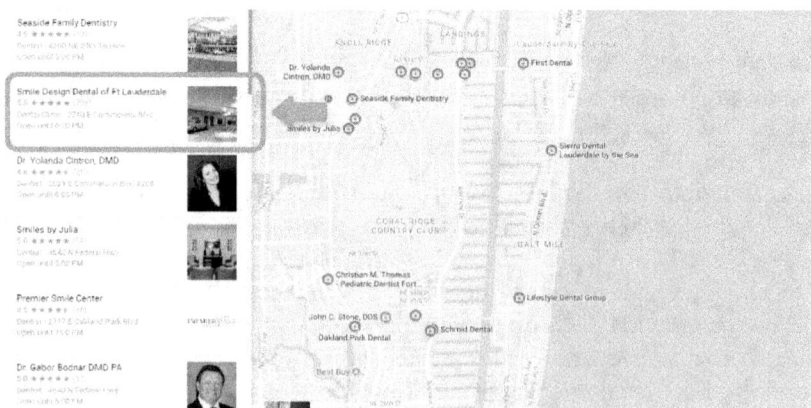

Conclusion

This is the end of the case study, but it is really only the beginning of your dental practice's journey toward sustainable patient growth.

If you're ready to take the next step to grow your dental practice using a customized dental marketing strategy that works, schedule a complimentary call with our team at (800) 398-0979. We'd be happy to chat with you.

About Firegang

We're Firegang Dental Marketing and we're passionate about 3 things:

- **Empowering dentists to attract new patients by executing marketing strategies.**
- **Creating real, measurable results so you know your practice is meeting its goals.**
- **Giving dentists the freedom to grow their practices, reclaim their time and their lives back**

Our clients are our first priority, and we're always looking for the latest dental marketing techniques to use in order to help dentists reach their practice goals.

Over the past 10+ years we've developed a full 360-degree dental marketing strategy that includes a conversion optimized website, Dental SEO, paid traffic campaigns on Google and Facebook, reputation marketing, and reviews. This approach is currently generating over 3,000 new patients per month for our clients.

We're looking for the best dental practices who are ready to partner with us, who want to take advantage of the growing opportunities digital advertising brings to produce new patients.

If you're ready to take the next step to grow your practice using a customized dental marketing strategy that works, click below to schedule a complimentary call with our team, we'd be happy to chat with you.

Make the one call that could change your life forever. Get in touch with our team at (800) 398-0979 and start growing your dental practice today.

ABOUT THE AUTHOR

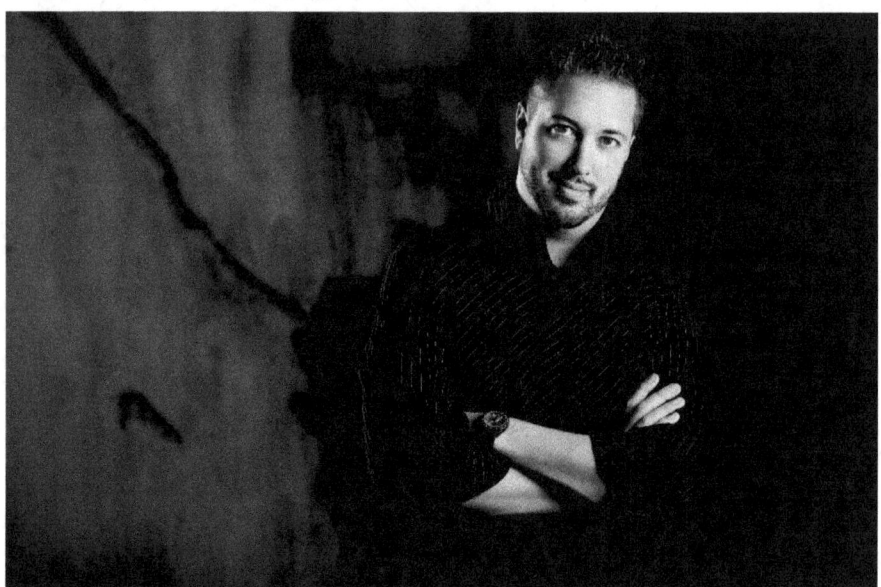

About Adam Zilko

Adam Zilko is a digital marketing expert, best selling author, and the founder and owner of Firegang Dental Marketing. Adam is known for his unique ability to help dental experts identify the best tools and techniques for attaining greater online visibility and attracting high-value patients for life.

Digital Marketing Expert

Adam has worked with thousands of dental professionals the world over, from single practices to multi-practice Dental Service Organizations (DSOs). Adam's knowledge and experience have contributed to some of the most successful dental web campaigns in operation today.

Adam is known for his ability to help dental experts set themselves apart online, improve their online reputations, and grow their practices with proven strategies that attract today's web-savvy dental prospects.

Owner & Founder of Firegang Dental Marketing

Along with his company, Firegang Dental Marketing, which he scaled from a simple startup to a multi-million-dollar company, Adam has successfully crafted highly-effective web presences for dental professionals around the country, and he's been able to deliver to those doctors more dental leads, improved sales, boosts in revenue and consistent practice growth each and every time.

An In-Depth Dental Marketing Approach

Adam and Firegang take an innovative, 360° dental marketing approach, which is nearly unheard of in the industry. Whereas most marketing companies remain solely web-focused, Firegang combines online and offline efforts to create a comprehensive dental patient attraction system.

The idea behind this method of marketing is based on Adam's philosophy of the buyer's journey, which acts as a multi-directional path that can cross channels with immense complexity.

Prospective patients may conduct a Google search, click on a Facebook Ad, visit the website, and these touchpoints may occur days, sometimes weeks apart. Each point along this path must be analyzed and fortified to ensure a secure and highly-performing dental web campaign from start to finish.

Real Dental Marketing Results

Adam has honed his knowledge of dental and digital marketing over years of managing hands-on business relationships with dentists, orthodontists, periodontists, dental surgeons, and DSOs the world over. The web and inter-office optimization techniques he and Firegang employ are based on measurable and substantial results.

Born and raised in Anchorage Alaska and residing in the Pacific Northwest, Adam is known as one of the premier dental and digital marketers in North America. He has earned hundreds of millions of dollars for his clients and continues to help dental professionals grow their practices and attain their lofty business goals to this day.

www.ingramcontent.com/pod-product-compliance
Lightning Source LLC
Chambersburg PA
CBHW052145220526
45471CB00004B/1531